MANUAL OF EQUINE DENTISTRY

Tom Allen, DVM, IAED/C
Private Practice
Patterson, Missouri

Christine King, BVSc, MACVSc (eq med), MVetClinStud
Consulting Editor
Cary, North Carolina

Dawn Sperry-Allen
Illustrator
Patterson, Missouri

with 300 illustrations

with 78 color plates

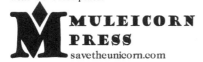

MULEICORN PRESS
savetheunicorn.com

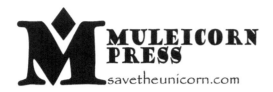
savetheunicorn.com

MANUAL OF EQUINE DENTISTRY   9780615229072

NOTICE

Veterinary medicine is an ever-changing field. Standard safety precautions must be followed, but as new research and clinical experience broaden our knowledge, changes in treatment and drug therapy may become necessary or appropriate. Readers are advised to check the most current product information provided by the manufacturer of each drug to be administered to verify the recommended dose, the method and duration of administration, and contraindications. It is the responsibility of the licensed veterinarian, relying on experience and knowledge of the patient, to determine dosages and the best treatment for each individual patient. Neither the publisher nor the author assumes any liability for any injury and/or damage to persons or property arising from this publication.

Library of Congress Cataloging-in-Publication Data
Allen, Tom, 1947-
    Manual of equine dentistry/Tom Allen.
       p. cm.
    Includes bibliographical references and index.
    ISBN 9780615229072
    1. Horses--Diseases. 2. Veterinary dentistry. I. Title.
SF959.M66A58 2003
636.1'08976--dc21

                               2003042150

Publishing Director: Linda Duncan
Acquisitions Editor: Liz Fathman
Developmental Editor: Jolynn Gower
Publishing Services Manager: Linda McKinley
Project Manager: Jennifer Furey
Designer 1st printing: Julia Dummitt
Designer 2nd printing: Elaine Lanmon
Cover Design 1st printing: MW Design
Cover Design 2nd printing: Dawn Sperry-Allen
Printed in the United States of America
Last digit is the print number: 9 8 7 6 5 4 3 2

CONTRIBUTORS

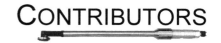

Tony Basile, IAED/Ex
El Dorado Hills, California

Michael Boero, DVM
Mahomet, Illinois

John Causey, IAED/Ex
Altuna, Florida

Michael H. Davis, DVM, IAED/C
Pearland, Texas

Scott K. Greene, DVM, IAED/CA
Sparks, Nevada

Dale Jeffrey, CP/EqD
Glenns Ferry, Idaho

Tom Johnson, DVM
Grass Lake, Michigan

Richard O. Miller, DVM, IAED/Ex
Cota De Caza, California

Carl Mitz, IAED/CA
Brenham, Texas

Lawrence A. Moriarity, EqDT-IAED/Ex
Ocala, Florida

Dennis Rach, DVM
Calgary, Alberta, Canada

William Schultze, IAED/C
Pittstown, New Jersey

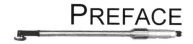

A friend, Frontster White, wrote this limerick. Frontster says he is our home state of Missouri's complement to Baxter Black.

To my non-veterinarian horse dental practitioner friends: Thanks! (To you and your predecessors for bringing it back.)

To my veterinary colleagues: Let's remember who brought it back and treat them honorably. And about this limerick: "Keep your sense of humor!"

We've been seeing many excellent articles about horse dentistry lately. Some of us may get the idea that horses will usually show definite symptoms when they need dentistry. Although it would seem reasonable for them to do so, the horse most often shows no sign whatsoever of even severe problems.

The Barrel Racer, The Roper, The Vet and the **Horse Dentist**
subtitle:
(Fat or Skinny, They've Problems A Many)
A Dental Limerick
By Frontster White

At the rodeo grounds that day,
The group that was there heard him say:
"Now, I'm no vet,
And they know lots, and yet:
Horse tooth care they've let get away!"

The man that stood there was saying
To all (even those beyond swaying)
That "Even if fat,
As sure as your hat,
In your horse's mouth sharp points are laying."

The crowd wasn't convinced, they were skeptical.
But rather than make a spectacle,
They just said, "Yeah sure"
But thought, "What manure!
Such talk will be his *debacle*."

For they knew horses working or idle,
If bothered in the feedbin or bridle
Would surely lose weight,
Or chew on the gate,
Or even just prance and sidle.

Then a barrel racer stepped up and said,
As up to the talker she led
A bay horse so shiny,
With quite a round hiney.
"If you find points here I'll turn red."

So onto the fat beast he did place
A speculum to show her the place
Where sharp points and crooks,
Like rows of meat hooks,
Were cutting the inside of Bay's face!

She turned red and started to gasp
"Please, sir, my Bay's teeth do rasp!
My vet said 'Go away,
His teeth are OK!'
But now his neck I will grasp!"

"I asked him to check the teeth
Of my gelding and now I seethe,
For even though fat,
Comfort's where it's at!
So Bay's fate to you I bequeath!"

Then a roper with a mount that was cheating,
Said "I'd druther take a beating
Than use this thin horse!"
(Doc checked him of course)
And said "OK, What's this horse been eating?"

He'd had his vet out to examine
The horse who was looking like famine.
And he had been told
"He's just getting old,
So to him 'complete feed' be crammin'."

The dentist looked in: "I pronounce:
This poor thing cannot gain an ounce
Til' we file those sharp peaks,
Way in the back there, in his cheeks
And then on each calf he will pounce!"

So the horse folks learned on that day
That the horse may stay chunky on hay
But he still may have hooks
(And….. this ain't in the books):
He won't gripe 'cause that's just his way!

Tom Allen
(alias Frontster White)

ACKNOWLEDGMENTS

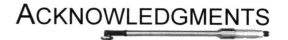

My understanding of equine dentistry has been gathered from many sources, including my colleagues in the International Association of Equine Dentistry (IAED) and my veterinary colleagues who have provided continuing education through the American Association of Equine Practitioners (AAEP). I particularly want to acknowledge the contributions of the following individuals, both to my education and to the advancement of the field of equine dentistry: Dale Jeffrey, Lawrence A. Moriarity, Carl Mitz, Tony Basile, and Drs. Gordon James Baker, Jack Easley, and W.L. Scrutchfield.

As I was researching material for this book, I was impressed by the fact that a span of 90 years passed between two seminal works on equine dentistry: *Animal Dentistry and Diseases of the Mouth* by Dr. Louis Merilliat, published in 1906 and *Equine Dentistry: the Theory and Practice of Equine Dental Maintenance* by Dale Jeffrey, published in 1996.

This fact highlights two key points about the field of equine dentistry. First, the dearth of information and advancements for much of the twentieth century is indicative of the attitude held by the majority of veterinary educators (and, sadly, many practicing veterinarians) toward equine dental care during that time. Second, we owe much of our current understanding of equine dental principles and practice to individuals outside the veterinary profession.

Fortunately, both situations have changed in recent years. We are now seeing many more publications and educational offerings by and for both veterinarians and equine dental technicians wanting to practice a higher standard of equine dentistry. To the individuals within and outside the veterinary profession who have continued to practice and teach a higher standard of equine dental care, thank you for your tireless efforts!

HOW TO USE THIS BOOK

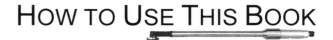

This book is intended as a practical guide to performing thorough dentistry in horses. It is written for veterinarians, veterinary students, and equine dental technicians. This manual is intended to pick up where formal education leaves off, so I have assumed that the reader has a basic understanding of equine oral and dental anatomy and is familiar with basic dental procedures such as hand floating. Anatomical diagrams are included in the text.

Only those procedures that can be performed in the field are included in this manual. For conditions requiring radiographic evaluation or surgery under general anesthesia, the reader is referred to other texts such as *Dentistry* (Veterinary Clinics of North America—Equine Practice, 14:2, Philadelphia, 1998, Saunders) and *Equine Dentistry* (G.J. Baker and K.J. Easley [editors], Philadelphia, 1999, Saunders).

For the most part, this manual comprises my understanding of equine dental structure and function, descriptions of how I perform specific dental procedures, and my rationale for the approach I use. My two main sources of knowledge and inspiration are (1) the numerous highly skilled and experienced equine dental technicians and veterinarians who have generously shared with me their knowledge of equine dentistry and (2) my equine patients, from whom I have learned and continue to learn so much.

However, I freely acknowledge that there are other ways of achieving the same goals of improved comfort, masticatory efficiency, performance, and longevity. I encourage the reader to seek out and learn from some of the many veterinarians and equine dental technicians who are practicing excellent equine dentistry across the United States and the rest of the world. Contributions from some of these individuals round out this manual and add considerably to its usefulness.

The first three chapters of this manual address the practicalities of incorporating thorough equine dentistry into an existing practice or business. The following four chapters describe examination of the horse's oral cavity and dental arcades, common dental abnormalities the practitioner can expect to find in practice, routine corrective or prophylactic procedures, and some specialized or selective procedures.

Rather than going straight to the chapter on performing routine procedures, I encourage the reader to review the preceding chapters to gain a better understanding of how common dental abnormalities develop and why they are a problem for the horse. The approach to correcting these abnormalities will then become clearer.

The book ends with a chapter on dental procedures in miniature horses and a chapter on continuing education resources. It is my hope that this book will inspire you to practice a higher standard of equine dentistry and continue to learn and advance this important field of equine health care.

Tom Allen, DVM, IAED/C

CONTENTS

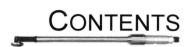

TOM ALLEN

MANUAL OF
EQUINE
DENTISTRY

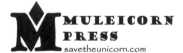
MULEICORN
PRESS
savetheunicorn.com

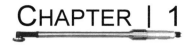

CHAPTER 1

Incorporating Equine Dentistry Into Your Practice

Tom Allen, John Causey, Michael H. Davis

WHY UPGRADE YOUR DENTISTRY SKILLS?

Dental disorders are a common problem in horses (Color Plate 1). In a slaughterhouse survey in which the heads of 500 horses and foals were examined, 80% had evidence of dental disease or other oral pathologic conditions.[1] Problems identified included sharp enamel points with associated buccal mucosal inflammation, ulceration, and fibrosis; abnormal wear leading to wave, shear, or step mouth formations; periodontal disease; missing teeth with consequent malocclusions; tooth fractures; polyodontia; bite abnormalities; and maleruptions. I see a similar incidence and range of dental disorders in my equine dentistry practice.

Despite the prevalence of dental problems in horses, dentistry is an area of equine health care that has largely been neglected by the veterinary profession—so much so that veterinarians are now scrambling to catch up to the level of knowledge and skill demonstrated by many conscientious and experienced equine dental technicians. Most equine veterinarians agree that dentistry is an integral part of equine preventive and therapeutic care and should be one of the services a general equine practice offers its clients. However, the tightly packed curricula of veterinary colleges leave little room for formal or practical training in this important area of equine practice. As a result, most veterinarians graduate from veterinary school with scant knowledge and few practical skills in equine dentistry.

There are at least four basic reasons for upgrading your knowledge and skills in equine dentistry and incorporating a higher standard of dentistry into your practice:

1. Dental problems can compromise a horse's health and well-being (Color Plate 2).
2. Dental problems can adversely affect a horse's performance and productivity.
3. Providing a higher standard of equine dentistry is a valuable service to your clients (Color Plate 3).
4. Providing a higher standard of equine dentistry adds to your practice income (Color Plate 4).

Health and Well-Being

Because horses use their teeth to prehend and masticate food, and because the teeth, gums, and other structures in the oral cavity are well supplied with blood and lymphatic vessels and sensory nerves, it is reasonable to surmise that dental disorders can adversely affect a horse's health and well-being. Unfortunately, this aspect of equine dentistry has not been widely studied.

Based on observation,[2] possible consequences of dental disease in horses include the following (Color Plates 5 and 6):
- Head shaking and facial pain
- Difficulty prehending and/or masticating food

- Reluctance to eat
- Degenerative joint disease of the temporomandibular joint(s) (TMJ)
- Oral ulceration
- Weight loss
- Digestive disturbances (e.g., choke, colic, diarrhea)
- Premature demise

Dental disorders can also cause bitting difficulties or affect athletic performance in other ways. These problems are discussed in the section on performance and productivity (Color Plate 7).

Masticatory Comfort and Efficiency

The most common dental problem I find in adult horses is sharp enamel points on the perimeter of the occlusal surfaces of the cheek teeth. Ulceration of the buccal mucosa is often found adjacent to these enamel points in the upper arcades. It hardly requires a scientific study to conclude that impingement of the soft tissues by these sharp enamel points can cause pain and thus may interfere with mastication to some degree.

Quidding (dropping partially chewed wads of grass or hay from the mouth) and weight loss are among the recognized symptoms of dental disease in horses,[2-5] and at least one study has shown an improvement in feed intake and weight gain following correction of dental abnormalities in horses.[6] I have observed cases in which horses gained weight after dental correction, although in my experience sharp enamel points are rarely the sole reason for weight loss or quidding.

Ralston, Foster, and Divers et al[7] conducted a feeding trial in which feed digestibility was evaluated before and after two common dental procedures: routine float (reduction of sharp enamel points and premolar hooks), and performance float (routine float plus smoothing of the buccal, palatal, and lingual ridges of the cheek teeth; removal of the transverse ridges from the occlusal surfaces of the cheek teeth; and rounding of the second premolars to produce a "bit seat"). Overall, feed digestibility was not affected by either procedure, although apparent digestibility of crude protein and fiber was reduced by the performance float when the table angle of the cheek teeth was greater than 80 degrees relative to the vertical axis of the teeth (i.e., when the occlusal surface was leveled).

Some detractors of thorough dentistry have used this study to prove that routine floating is of little advantage to the horse. However, the horses used in this study had only minor dental abnormalities. None had missing or fractured teeth, large hooks, ramps, wave mouth, steps, appreciable periodontal disease, or other serious dental pathologic conditions that I commonly find in my first-time patients.

An interesting phenomenon noted by some authors,[8] and one I have observed in my practice, is the presence of severe oral pathologic findings in apparently healthy horses in reasonably good body condition (Fig. 1-1). This fact, too, has been used by some to support their belief that dental disorders in horses are overinflated in importance. However, in my opinion this phenomenon relates more to the fact that many domesticated horses are overfed relative to their caloric needs: a horse that would probably lose body condition "in the wild" often is able to maintain its body weight on a highly digestible, easily assimilated, calorie-dense, man-made diet. In my opinion, the potential for oral pain caused by dental overgrowths is sufficient justification for recommending thorough dental care on a regular basis.

Wilewski and Rubin[9] reported that removing sharp enamel points from the cheek teeth and correcting any dental malalignments improved the masticatory efficiency in a group of Saddlebred horses in training. The mastication score was based on the amount of grain spillage, the time taken to finish eating, and observation of any abnormal behavior (e.g., head tilt, "yawning") while eating. Although an admittedly subjective assessment, this simple field study documented what I have found in many of my patients: removing any hindrances to mastication and balancing the dental arcades improves the horse's masticatory comfort and efficiency.

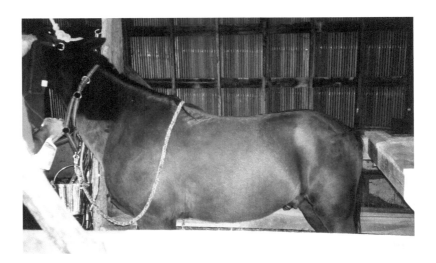

Figure 1-1. **A**, A healthy looking horse with good body condition.

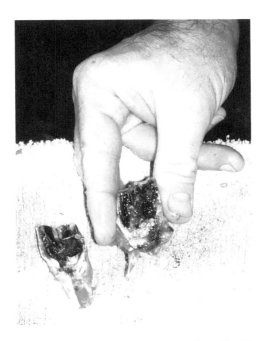

Figure 1-1. B, Dental examination revealed that this "healthy" horse had two sagittally fractured upper 9s.

Infections

Disease involving the roots of the third through sixth cheek teeth in horses is a well-documented cause of infection in the maxillary sinuses and sometimes, by extension, other paranasal sinuses.[10,11] Whether routine dentistry would decrease the incidence of this problem remains to be determined. It can be argued that thorough oral examination on a regular basis, as part of routine dental care, might identify a diseased tooth early enough for treatment to prevent apical infection and secondary sinusitis. Certainly, regular dental care is important in preserving efficient mastication following extraction of a diseased cheek tooth.

In human and small animal dentistry, bacteremia associated with periodontal disease is well documented and has been implicated in the development of systemic disease, including glomerulonephritis, pyelonephritis, bacterial endocarditis and myocarditis, hepatitis, and fever of unknown origin.[12] One study in dogs found an association between the severity of periodontal disease and the severity of histopathologic changes in the kidney, liver, and myocardium.[12] Kirkland, Marretta, and Inoue[1] noted that the frequency and severity of periodontal disease increased with age in horses. Assuming that bacteremia occurs in horses with severe periodontal disease as it does in other species, periodontitis could be an important contributor to organ disease and the premature demise of older horses (Color Plate 8).

Management Factors

Another factor that can adversely affect the health and longevity of older horses is the outlay of time and money required to appropriately feed horses that have lost, worn, maloccluded, or otherwise poorly functioning teeth. Some horse owners are unwilling or unable to bear the responsibility of managing these horses properly.

Kirkland, Marretta, and Inoue[1] concluded that the higher incidence of periodontal disease and abnormalities of wear found in older horses is the culmination of a lifetime of dental neglect. By implication, regular dental care may prevent, or at least minimize, the pathologic changes that result from abnormal wear and may thus minimize the effects of aging (Fig. 1-2A).

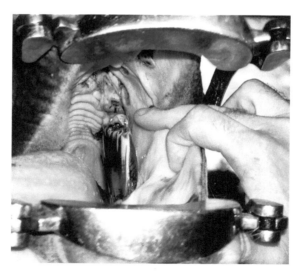

Figure 1-2. A, 19-year-old gelding with unopposed 306 and 307 and severe ulcerations into the nasal passage.

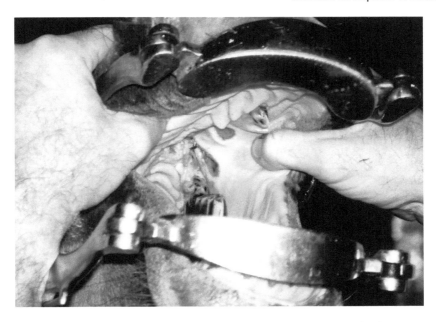

Figure 1-2. B, The same horse with severe life threatening malocclusions.

Performance and Productivity

In horses that are ridden or driven, dental abnormalities that cause pain (e.g., sharp enamel points) or that limit the rostral-caudal movement of the mandible (e.g., hooks or ramps) can affect performance in a number of ways. Manifestations variably include bit chewing, tongue lolling (hanging the tongue out the side of the mouth), resistance to the bit, head tossing, hanging or tipping the head to one side, running out, refusal to stop, reluctance or inability to perform maneuvers that require poll flexion, tail wringing, stiff gait, and even lameness.[3,5,13,14] Failure to recognize dental disorders as the cause of these behaviors in a young horse can create training problems that last a lifetime.

In the study reported by Wilewski and Rubin,[9] athletic performance and responsive-ness to the trainer's aids were improved in all 20 horses after initial dental work (which included removal of sharp enamel points and correction of any dental malalignments). An improvement was noted even in horses described by the trainer as having a "good mouth" before the dental work was performed. Creating a bit seat (rounding the rostral margin of the first cheek teeth) further improved athletic performance in 60% of horses. Again, this field study mirrors what I have found in my practice: resolving dental conditions that cause pain or that interfere with normal function can substantially improve the horse's performance.

In breeding animals, dental problems that affect mastication (e.g., excessive or abnormal wear, premature tooth loss) can negatively affect productivity by decreasing feed efficiency and increasing the time and expense required to keep an animal in acceptable body condition. For example, special diets and feeding regimens may be required to maintain breeding animals with uncorrectable dental problems.

Serving Your Clients' Needs

Based on the impact of dental disorders on health and performance, providing a high standard of dental care is a valuable service to your patients and thus to your clients. The value of this service to a particular patient may be therapeutic (i.e., identification and correction of existing abnormalities) or prophylactic (i.e., regular examinations and correction of any minor abnormalities before they become a significant problem).

As the growing number of articles in equestrian magazines and on the Internet educate horse owners and trainers about the importance of dentistry to their horses' health and performance, the demand for high-quality equine dental care will continue to increase. The adage "if you don't, someone else will" is apt when it comes to equine dentistry. Consider whether you want your clients to use a dental technician or veterinarian of uncertain experience and competence, or to call you to fulfill their horses' dentistry needs.

Even if you do not have the time or the interest to include a full range of equine dentistry services in your veterinary practice, being able to perform a thorough oral examination and recognize common dental problems, and understanding what is required to correct these problems provides a valuable service to your clients. For problems you feel are beyond your scope (whether of time, equipment, or experience), referring the patient to a colleague or enlisting the services of an equine dental technician who is better equipped to manage the problem is also a service to your patients and to your clients.

Profitability

Providing a higher standard of equine dentistry can add to your practice income. As Fig. 1-3 illustrates, the three key components to increasing your practice income from equine dentistry are these:

1. Increasing client demand for thorough dentistry
2. Charging a fee that reflects your knowledge and skill
3. Improving your work efficiency

Although the following comments chiefly pertain to veterinarians in equine or large animal practice, the same principles apply to equine dental technicians who want to expand their practices.

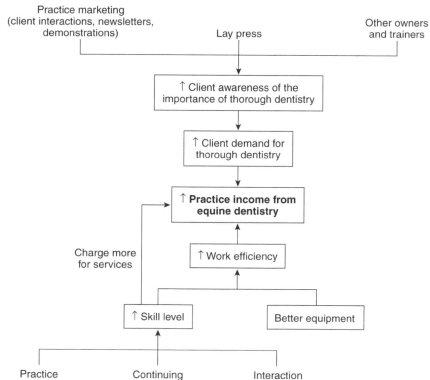

Figure 1-3. Increasing your practice income from equine dentistry.

Increasing Client Demand

Creating or increasing the demand for your dentistry skills among your equine clients is simple. Articles in the lay press and conversations with other horse owners and trainers are already doing some of the work for you. Conversations you have with clients at routine visits (e.g., annual or semiannual preventive health care visits), short articles in practice newsletters, and demonstrations at open days or other client education gatherings are just a few of the ways you can make current and prospective clients aware of the advantages of thorough equine dentistry. Marketing equine dentistry is discussed further in the next section.

Charging Appropriately

Provided you charge a fee that adequately compensates you for your time and reflects your level of education and experience, upgrading your dental skills and equipment will increase your practice income, even if you perform only a handful of routine dental procedures per week. It can also make the practice of equine dentistry more interesting and enjoyable, which is a less tangible but no less important reward.

There are two basic approaches to setting up a fee schedule. One is to charge the "going rate"—the average fee charged by other practitioners (whether veterinarians or equine dental technicians) in your area for that particular procedure. The other approach is to determine approximately how long a particular procedure takes you to complete and set a fee that adequately compensates you for your time, equipment costs, and the skill required to perform the procedure. Although keeping fees competitive is a consideration for many practitioners, it is nonetheless important to set fees that generate sufficient revenue to allow you to stay in business and enjoy your work.

I incorporated both approaches when setting my fee schedule. I used the going rate as a starting point and developed a range of fees for the procedures I commonly perform. By using a range, rather than a set fee, I can charge a little more if the procedure proves to be more difficult or takes longer than usual in a particular patient, while still giving clients an accurate estimate of what they will be charged.

The initial examination, sedation (and reversal, if used), dental examination and charting, and specific procedures can be charged separately (i.e., itemized) or they can be bundled together in some way. If all recommended dental corrections are performed during the visit, I bundle the examination, charting, and initial sedation and reversal charges into the procedure fee. Additional sedation and other medications administered or prescribed are charged separately. If the client elects not to have the recommended dental corrections performed during that visit, I itemize the individual procedures, charging a separate fee for the initial examination, sedation and reversal, dental examination and charting, and whatever dental work is performed. In addition to the examination fee, I charge a farm call or set-up fee when I work on fewer than five horses at one location.

Improving Work Efficiency

Improving your work efficiency is basically a function of increasing your skill level and using equipment that makes the job quicker and easier. Increasing your skill level is accomplished through practice and education, whether at continuing education courses, by reading books and articles on equine dentistry, or through interactions with colleagues who perform a high standard of equine dentistry (see Chapter 9). Tools and equipment are discussed in Chapter 2; performing specific procedures expediently is discussed in Chapter 6.

MARKETING DENTISTRY IN YOUR PRACTICE

Marketing equine dentistry begins with client education. By educating horse owners and trainers about the advantages of thorough equine dentistry, veterinarians and other equine dental practitioners expand the market for their services. With clients who are already aware of the benefits and perhaps have had to resort to seeking quality equine dental care elsewhere, you reinforce their faith in your concern for their horses and in your ability to provide comprehensive dental care. (Fig. 1-4)

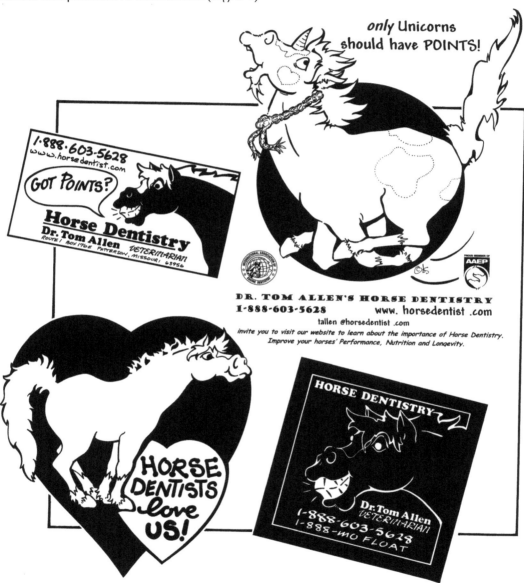

Figure 1-4. Sample promotional material that I use to advertise dental services. (*Horse Dentistry, Copyright 1996, Dawn Sperry-Allen; Got Points? Copyright 1997, Dawn Sperry-Allen; Horse Dentists Love Us, Copyright 1998, Dawn Sperry-Allen; Only Unicorns Should Have Points, Copyright 2002, Dawn Sperry-Allen.*)

In contrast to some aspects of equine health care, dental care is relatively easy to promote. Allowing the owner or trainer to look, and perhaps even feel, in the horse's mouth during your initial examination can be a powerful educational and marketing tool. For many horse owners, even seasoned owners and trainers, the first time they see into the depths of their horses' mouths is a dramatic experience. Usually the first thing that impresses them is how far back into the mouth the cheek teeth extend. Having dental abnormalities pointed out is even more memorable (although somewhat repulsive to some owners). Some of the more dramatic "surprises" that may be found hiding behind the horse's lips include the following:

- Canine teeth that are 1 inch or more in height and surprisingly sharp, often accompanied by telltale lacerations or scarring on the ventral surface of the tongue (Color Plate 9)
- Large hooks on the upper 6s (upper first cheek teeth) that may be so long that they carve out notches in the bars of the mandible (Color Plate 10)
- Ramps on the lower 6s (lower first cheek teeth) that are so tall they have created ulcerations on the hard palate or have completely overpowered the upper 6s, grinding them down to stumps (Color Plate 11)
- Waves (undulating tables on the cheek teeth arcades) of such severity that the upper cheek teeth are worn away and the patient is chewing with root fragments (Color Plate 12)
- Sagittally fractured upper 9 (upper fourth cheek tooth), with one half of the tooth diverging toward the hard palate and the other half leaning out and creating deep ulcerations in the buccal mucosa (Color Plate 13)
- Ramps on lower 11s (lower sixth cheek teeth) that are so long they create holes in the roof of the mouth just caudal to the last molars or they grind down part of the corresponding upper molars (see Fig. 5-31)

What often amazes owners and trainers is that these gross abnormalities can be present in horses that outwardly appear normal (good body condition, good appetite, well mannered) and are seemingly problem-free. However, if seeing such pathologic conditions in their horses' mouths fails to convince them, seeing the difference in the horse's attitude and performance following corrective procedures usually sells them on the importance of regular, thorough dental care (Color Plate 14).

Countering Misconceptions

Articles on equine dental care have become common in equestrian magazines over the past few years. Although this exposure is a valuable asset toward the goal of incorporating quality dental care into veterinary practices, misconceptions remain and must be addressed when marketing equine dentistry to existing or prospective clients.

The Inadequate Check

A common recommendation made by the authors of such articles (whether veterinarian or other professional) is to have the horse's teeth checked every 6 to 12 months. Although this recommendation, in itself, may be sound, it has resulted in the perpetuation of dental neglect because the concept of "checking a horse's teeth" is not defined.

Too often the "check" has consisted of a practitioner feeling the outer edges of the upper cheek teeth along the sides of the horse's face or sticking a finger in the horse's mouth and feeling the buccal edges of the first one or two upper cheek teeth and declaring that, "the teeth are OK," if no excessively sharp points are found (Fig. 1-5). With this approach, extensive dental pathologic conditions can develop and may progress to an untreatable stage, despite the conscientious owner having had the horse's teeth regularly checked, as advised. Thus one key component of client education is making clear, in word and action, what constitutes a proper dental examination. (Examination of the oral cavity is described in Chapter 4.)

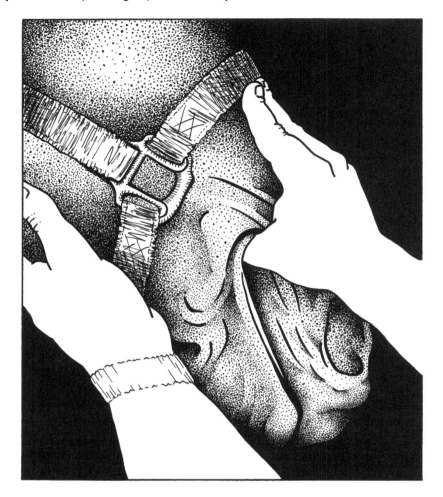

Figure 1-5. An inadequate dental check.

Signs of Dental Disease

Many articles on equine dental care, both in equestrian magazines and veterinary publications, list signs that indicate the presence of dental disease or the need for dental care. These lists are accurate, in that any horse exhibiting those signs is likely to be suffering from dental disease; and they can be helpful in directing an owner or trainer of a horse showing such symptoms to seek dental care for the horse. However, these lists can also be misleading if the author does not make clear that *the absence of those signs does not mean the absence of dental disease*. It is a fallacy that horses with dental problems always, or even often, exhibit easily recognizable symptoms (Fig. 1-6).

It is important to impress upon horse owners and trainers that lists of observed behaviors cannot be relied on to determine the need for dental care. *You cannot know what is going on in a horse's mouth unless you look*. And informed judgments or decisions concerning the horse's dental health cannot be made until a thorough oral examination has been performed.

Follow-Up

As in many aspects of business, follow-up is important in marketing equine dentistry in your practice. As discussed later, providing a written report is a valuable marketing tool. Sending reminder notices to clients when it is time for them to schedule routine dental work is also a useful practice. With business software streamlining recordkeeping in the office, sending out reminders based on your specific recommendations for each horse is a simple and effective practice-building exercise (Color Plate 15).

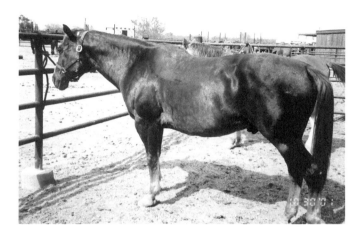

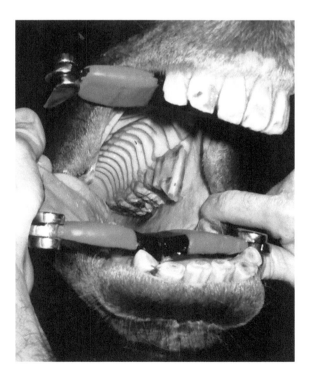

Figure 1-6. A, This horse is outwardly healthy but his mouth indicates otherwise. **B,** The same "outwardly healthy" horse has a severe parrot mouth and upper 6 hooks with lower 11 ramps.

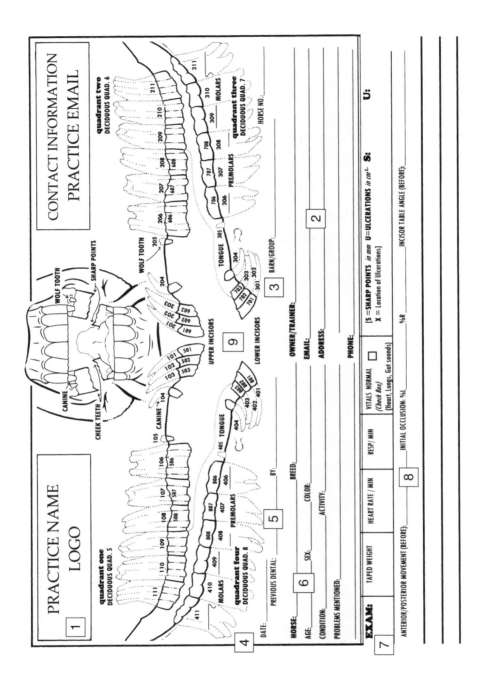

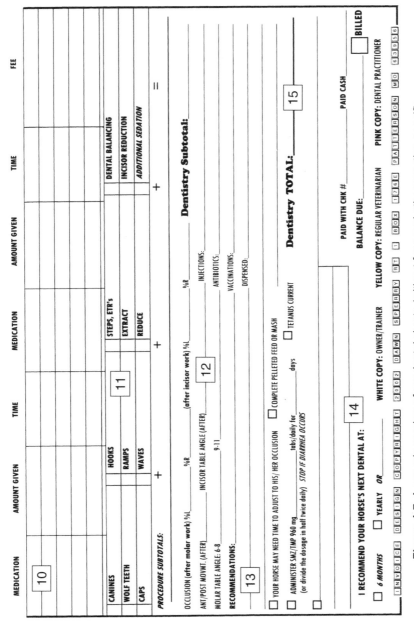

Figure 1-7. A generic version of my dental charts (without fees and other practice-specific information). (Copyright 2001, Dawn Sperry-Allen.)

RECORDKEEPING

A standard patient record, including signalment and pertinent medical history (see item 6 in the following list), should be made for every horse examined, even if the procedure was limited to a brief oral examination. A dental chart should also be completed for every horse examined. Another means of documenting oral abnormalities is to take a photograph, although photography should not be used in place of the dental chart. Finally, before sedating a horse and performing any dental procedures, it is prudent to discuss the planned procedure with the owner or agent and perhaps have that person sign a consent form.

Dental Chart

The dental chart I currently use is shown in Fig. 1-7. I use the modified Triadan system for identifying the individual teeth; this system is used throughout this manual. When formulating a dental chart for use in your practice, the following items are important:
1. Name and contact details of the practitioner—include both the practitioner's name and the business name (if applicable), physical or postal address of the business, telephone and fax number(s), e-mail address, and website address (if applicable).
2. Name and contact details of the owner—include this information even if the work was requested by a trainer or other agent.
3. Location—state the location of the facility at which the work was performed, if different from the owner's address above.
4. Date—give the date of the current examination.
5. Dental history—include the date of the previous dental examination, name of the practitioner who performed the last examination, nature of any dental work done at that time, and other pertinent information.
6. Signalment and medical history—state the horse's name, breed, age, gender, color, estimated body weight, body condition, use, and any problems reported by the owner, rider, or trainer.
7. Physical examination findings—(see Chapter 4).
8. Oral examination findings—detail findings and list indices that are graded or measured, such as the angles of the incisor and molar tables, the amount of rostral-caudal movement of the mandible, and the percentage of molar occlusion (see Chapter 4).
9. Dentition chart—use a diagram that shows the typical adult equine dentition from the craniocaudal view (i.e., incisors viewed from the front of the horse) and from both the left and right sides; use appropriate labeling to identify the individual teeth.
10. Medication(s) given—list drug name, dosage, and route and time(s) of administration for each drug given (sedatives, analgesics, reversal agents, antiinflammatory medications, antibiotics); list details for any drugs left with the client for continued treatment.
11. Dental procedure(s) performed—allow sufficient space to detail the procedures performed during the current visit, as a reference for future dental visits.
12. Postprocedure remarks—I use this section to record the angle of the incisor and molar tables, rostral-caudal movement of the mandible, the percentage of molar occlusion, and any other observations made following the dental work.
13. Recommendations to owner/agent—leave sufficient space or write prompts that detail feeding instructions, training recommendations (e.g., __ days off before resuming training), and specific instructions for any medications dispensed.
14. Date of next dental examination—depending on the circumstances, give either a specific date or a time frame (e.g., revisit in 6 months).
15. Fees—include charges for examination, medication(s), and dental procedures. I list a range of fees for common procedures on the dental chart; this list acts as a prompt when I am totaling the charges at the end of the visit.

The dental record I use is a triplicate form, printed on carbonless paper, with one copy for the owner, one for the referring veterinarian or trainer, and one for my records. It serves as a detailed record of the condition of the patient's mouth both before and after the dental work was performed, the nature of any corrective procedures, quantitative results of these procedures (e.g., table angles, percent occlusion), medications administered, and recommendations made for continuing care and revisit. This record can be invaluable if questions ever arise about the condition of the patient before or immediately after treatment.

While conducting the dental examination, pointing out each item entered on the dental chart by allowing the client to look inside the horse's mouth is an excellent way of educating clients and convincing them of the need for any corrections you recommend. Allowing the client to inspect the horse's mouth again, after the dental work is completed, is a graphic way of demonstrating the difference your work has made. Together with a copy of the dental chart, this inspection is a powerful educational and marketing tool.

Camera

Photography is an excellent means of documenting the state of the teeth and oral soft tissues before and after corrective procedures are performed. Photographs of the dental structures may simply be used for routine recordkeeping (i.e., as part of the horse's dental record), but they are particularly valuable as legal documentation should a client or other dental practitioner make an accusation at any time. In addition, by routinely photographing the mouth of every horse examined, a practitioner may build up an extensive catalog of dental abnormalities, which is a valuable educational resource.

Digital cameras are ideal for this purpose, because on most models the photograph can be viewed immediately and the shot repeated if necessary. Good-quality photographs of the more rostral structures (incisors, canines, first few cheek teeth, tongue, bars, buccal mucosa just caudal to the commissures of the lips) are relatively easy to obtain. However, getting good photographs of the more caudal structures can be a challenge. Endoscopy (using either a flexible or rigid endoscope) is best suited for this purpose.

Informed Consent Form

Most legal experts recommend the use of a form on which the owner or agent (1) confirms that the risks of any recommended procedure(s) have been explained to them, and (2) consents, in writing, to the performance of the procedure(s) by the practitioner. Such forms may offer some protection for the individual providing the service in the event of any unforeseen injury to the horse or to the owner or assistant. Although a standard consent form for surgical procedures may suffice, it may be worth discussing the content and wording with an attorney before creating a consent form specifically for dental procedures.

REFERENCES

1. Kirkland KD, Marretta SM, Inoue OJ: Survey of equine dental disease and associated oral pathology. Proceedings of the Fortieth Annual Convention of the American Association of Equine Practitioners, Lexington, KY, 1994.
2. Knottenbelt DC: The systemic effects of dental disease. In Baker GJ, Easley J, editors: Equine dentistry, London, 1999, WB Saunders.
3. Baker GJ: Dental physical examination, Vet Clin North Am Equine Pract 14:247, 1998.
4. Crabill MR, Schumacher J: Pathophysiology of acquired dental diseases of the horse, Vet Clin North Am Equine Pract 14:291, 1998.
5. Dixon PM: Removal of equine dental overgrowths, Equine Vet Ed 2A:92, 2000.
6. Krusic L, Easley J, Pagan J et al: Influence of corrected teeth on daily food consumption and glucose availability in horses. Proceedings of the first Symposium on Horse Diseases, Radenci, Slovenia, 1995.
7. Ralston SL, Foster DL, Divers T et al: Effect of dental correction on feed digestibility in horses, Equine Vet J 33:390, 2001.
8. Brigham EJ, Duncanson GR: Case study of 100 horses presented to an equine dental technician in the UK, Equine Vet Ed 2A:84, 2000.
9. Wilewski KA, Rubin L: Bit seats: a dental procedure for enhancing performance of show horses, Equine Pract 21:16, 1999.
10. Tremaine WH, Dixon PM: A long-term study of 277 cases of equine sinonasal disease. I. Details of horses, historical, clinical and ancillary diagnostic findings, Equine Vet J 33:274, 2001.
11. Tremaine WH, Dixon PM: A long-term study of 277 cases of equine sinonasal disease. II. Treatments and results of treatments, Equine Vet J 33:283, 2001.
12. DeBowes LJ, Mosier D, Logan E et al: Association of periodontal disease and histologic lesions in multiple organs from 45 dogs, J Vet Dent 13:57, 1996.

13. Scoggins RD: Teeth and performance: a review of basic equine dentistry, Large Anim Vet 44:30, 1989.
14. Scoggins RD: Bits, bitting, and dentistry. Proceedings of the Forty-Seventh Annual Convention of the American Association of Equine Practitioners, Lexington, KY, 2001.

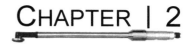

CHAPTER 2

Dental Tools and Equipment

William Schultze, Tom Allen, Carl Mitz, Tom Johnson

HAND TOOLS VERSUS POWER TOOLS

Power tools (motorized instruments) have become synonymous with thorough equine dentistry in the minds of many practitioners and horse owners (Color Plate 16). In fact, there is a tendency for veterinarians to view power tools as the standard for high-quality equine dentistry. But although some dental overgrowths are best managed using power tools, motorized equipment is not necessary to perform thorough dentistry. Power tools don't do a better job than hand tools; they simply make the same job easier on the practitioner.

Advantages of Hand Tools

Most dental procedures can be performed—and performed well—using hand tools alone (Fig. 2-1). In fact, there are several advantages to using hand tools over power tools:
- Hand tools are much less expensive to purchase, maintain, and replace.
- With hand tools, most procedures can be performed without sedation in the majority of patients.
- There is no possibility of thermal damage to the teeth when hand tools are used.
- Excessive reduction of crown height is much less likely than when power tools are used.
- There is less chance of inadvertently causing trauma to the oral tissues with hand tools.
- Electricity is not required with hand tools, so dental work can be performed at facilities that do not have a reliable power supply (e.g., run-in sheds, pastures).
- The practitioner has a better tactile sense when working with hand tools.
- With hand tools, less time is required to set up and pack up the equipment.

A few horses simply will not hold their heads still for power dental equipment, no matter how heavily they are sedated. Short of general anesthesia, hand tools may be the only option in these patients.

Sedation-Free Dentistry

Being able to perform dental procedures without sedation potentially has several advantages (Fig. 2-2):
- Less time is required for each patient (no waiting for sedation to have maximal effect and to be reversed).
- Less expense is incurred for the client (no cost for sedative, reversal agent, or injec- tion fee).

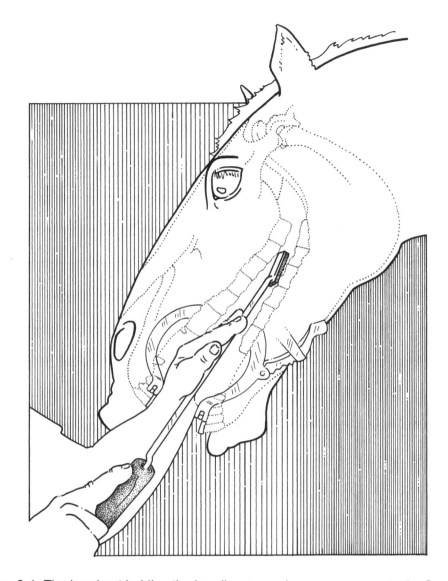

Figure 2-1. The hand not holding the handle can apply more pressure to the float. This patient's position is more normal than that of the patient in Color Plate 16, making use of hand floats easier and often not requiring sedation.

- Risks associated with sedation and intravenous injection (e.g., inadvertent injection into the carotid artery, leakage of drug outside the jugular vein, damage to the vessel wall) are eliminated.
- The horse can be fed or exercised immediately after the procedure, allowing improvements in mastication or behavior when ridden to be assessed right away, without the need for reversal agents.
- The horse can be moved or transported immediately after the procedure, without the need for reversal agents.
- Some owners do not want their horses sedated unless absolutely necessary; choosing not to sedate these horses can build your practice.
- Provided the horse is handled sensitively and dental procedures are performed with care, having the horse fully conscious allows it to become accustomed to the procedures,

thus more willing to tolerate them on subsequent visits.
- The horse's awareness of or response to pain is not masked, so there is less likelihood of inducing tissue trauma (because the unsedated patient will not tolerate a painful procedure).

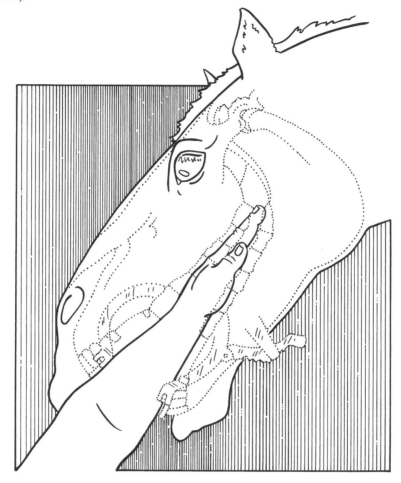

Figure 2-2. These areas may be blocked from vision by the tongue, so they must be felt with the fingertips (palm up for feeling the upper teeth).

There are, of course, situations in which administration of a sedative-analgesic drug or combination is necessary for the patient's comfort and cooperation.

Thermal Injury

Because of the speed at which the motorized burr, float, or disk rotates or oscillates on the surface of the tooth, there is the potential for power tools to generate sufficient friction to overheat the tooth and cause thermal damage to the vital tissues of the tooth. However, in our opinion the potential for thermal injury is negligible with proper technique: keeping the instrument moving over the tooth, rather than remaining in one place.

With some power dental tools, water is delivered to the head of the instrument during operation to flush away any debris and vaporized material. The water also cools the instrument and the tooth, which further reduces the risk of thermal injury.

Work Efficiency

Although set-up and pack-up times can be considerable when using power tools, motorized instruments can substantially shorten the time it takes to perform specific dental procedures (Color Plate 17). Motorized instruments also make dentistry easier on the practitioner's body. However, there are situations in which hand floating generally is faster and more efficient:

- When only one or two horses are to be done—it may take longer to set up and pack up the power tools than it takes to do the entire job with hand tools.
- When floating the teeth of young horses—young horses have softer teeth than older horses, and most have not had time to develop severe malocclusions.
- In horses that regularly receive thorough dental care—in most cases, these patients do not develop large overgrowths or other changes requiring removal of large amounts of tooth between visits.

Master Hand Tools First

Routine dental procedures should be mastered using hand floats before the practitioner advances to using motorized instruments (Color Plate 18). After becoming proficient with hand floating, safe and efficient use of power equipment is much easier to master. Learning to use power instruments should be a slow and careful process. A large amount of tooth can be removed very quickly and less-experienced practitioners tend to overfloat.

When using any power instrument, extreme care must be taken to avoid trauma to the soft tissues of the horse's mouth (tongue, gum, cheek, lips, and palate). It is best to use power instruments with a stationary guard to avoid soft tissue damage. Motorized equipment for equine dentistry may be electric or pneumatic. Specific instruments are discussed next.

PURCHASING EQUIPMENT

Carl Mitz and Tom Allen

Thorough equine dentistry requires more than a couple of dental floats and a bucket. Basic equipment should include a full-mouth speculum, a variety of carbide hand floats, dental extractors, dental probes, and a good light source. Motorized equipment may also be considered if dentistry is to become a significant portion of your practice.

The purchase of dental instruments is a considerable investment. It is well worth taking the time to research available instruments and manufacturers thoroughly before making a purchase. Buying the best quality instruments available is a worthwhile investment, because you should never need to replace these items in the normal course of practice. Whenever possible, purchase instruments made of good-quality stainless steel.

If possible, attend at least one trade show before purchasing dental instruments. Handle as many of the instruments and other equipment as you can to get a feel for them. Other ways of learning about the range, uses, and feel of the various equine dental instruments include attending equine dentistry workshops and spending some time with a colleague who routinely performs thorough equine dentistry. The instruments are an extension of your hand, so choose tools that feel comfortable to hold and use. Sources for equine dental instruments are listed in the Appendix (Fig. 2-3 and Color Plate 19).

Full-Mouth Speculum

Of all the instruments an equine dental practitioner should own, a full-mouth speculum is among the most important. The oral cavity cannot be thoroughly examined in the standing horse without using a full-mouth speculum. Also, working on the cheek teeth can be very difficult unless a full-mouth speculum is used to maximize visibility of, and access to, this part of the mouth.

There are two basic types of full-mouth speculum: McPherson and McAllen. The McPherson-type speculum (also known as the *Haussman gag*) has been around for 100 years and has changed very little in that time (Fig. 2-4). It provides excellent access to the oral cavity, although access to the buccal surfaces of the cheek teeth can be limited by the sides of the speculum. One way to maximize access is to use an attachment (an inverted U–shaped suspension bar) that sits over the bridge of the horse's nose and holds the sides of the speculum away from the horse's cheeks* (Fig. 2-5). Some newer models of McPherson speculum allow a wide range of jaw angle adjustment for better patient comfort.

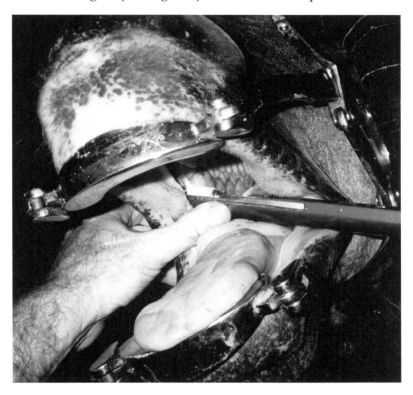

Figure 2-3. A guarded burr in use on a large upper 6 hook. Sometimes power equipment can make the work much easier on the patient and the practitioner.

The McAllen-type speculum allows better access to the buccal surfaces of the cheek teeth, which can be important when using motorized equipment on the cheek teeth arcades (see Fig. 2-2). However, the McAllen speculum is considerably larger and somewhat heavier than McPherson-type specula. To address this problem, at least one manufacturer now offers an aluminum McAllen-type speculum.*

When selecting a speculum of either type, buy one constructed of good-quality stainless steel (or heavy-duty aluminum for the McAllen speculum). Chrome specula tend to rust and flake, which makes them difficult to clean and decreases their durability. Full-mouth specula vary widely in price; ensure that the quality matches the price before purchasing any speculum.

Other Types of Specula

There are several other devices for holding the patient's mouth open (Fig. 2-6). Although some are useful, none provide the visibility and access of a full-mouth speculum; and some types can even be harmful to the horse. Spool gags consist of a metal coil that is fitted between the upper and lower cheek teeth arcades. These devices should be avoided because they concentrate the vertical forces generated by the masticatory muscles across just one or two pairs of teeth. If a horse bites down on a spool gag with sufficient force, the gag can fracture a tooth, particularly if the tooth is already compromised.

Wedge gags are safer than spool gags, particularly if they are constructed of a more "giving" material than metal. Owing to their shape, they distribute the vertical forces across several teeth, thus minimizing the risk of tooth fracture if the horse bites down on the gag with great force. However, both spool and wedge gags load the left and right TMJs unevenly when used singly. Whenever possible, wedge gags should be used in pairs, one for each side of the mouth.

There is a full-mouth speculum available that uses a crank or screw device to forcibly open the horse's jaws. In our opinion, this device has considerable potential for harm, because it is easy for the practitioner to open the horse's jaws wider than is comfortable for the horse, and thus place excessive strain on the TMJs, masticatory muscles, and the commissures of the lips. When fitting other types of full-mouth specula, the horse opens its mouth at the prompting of the practitioner. This simple action affords the practitioner the opportunity to assess the ability and willingness of the horse to open its mouth and the range of jaw angle the horse can comfortably accommodate.

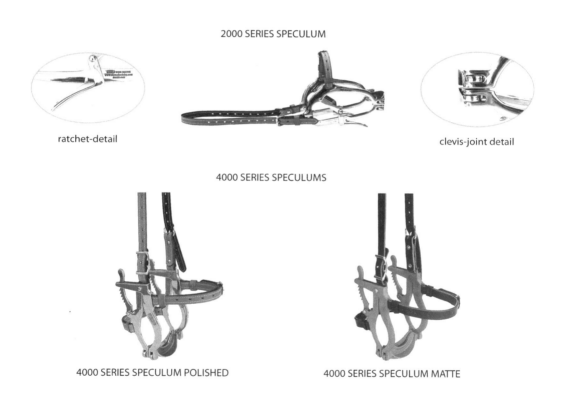

2000 SERIES SPECULUM

ratchet-detail

clevis-joint detail

4000 SERIES SPECULUMS

4000 SERIES SPECULUM POLISHED

4000 SERIES SPECULUM MATTE

Figure 2-4. Full-mouth speculum photos (McPherson-type). (Courtesy World Wide Equine, Inc., Glenns Ferry, Idaho)

Timer

Minimizing the time a patient's mouth is held open by a speculum is important for ensuring the patient's comfort and cooperation. Because it is easy to lose track of time when working, I use a kitchen timer, set for 10 minutes, to alert me that it is time to close the speculum and give the horse's jaws a 30- to 60-second rest. During the break time, I massage the horse's temporalis muscles. This simple technique has decreased the incidence and severity of postdentistry discomfort and inappetence in my patients (Fig. 2-7).

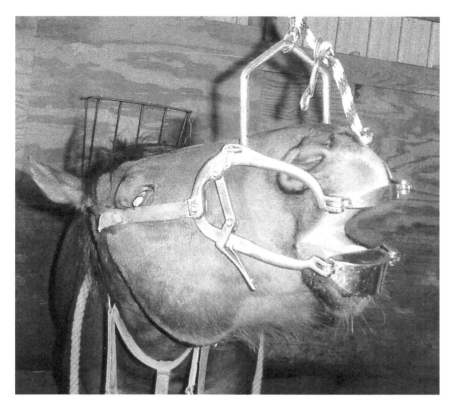

Figure 2-5. Speculum and inverted U-shaped suspension or spreader bar in use. Note snap on bar as safety link.

Light Source

Illumination of the oral cavity is very important in equine dentistry. The light source you use should be bright enough to illuminate the caudalmost structures in the oral cavity. When choosing a light source, consider candle power (intensity), weight, and cost. Although a good penlight with fresh batteries may be adequate, halogen lights are better choices, and are available as hand-held lights or headlamps. Head-mounted lamps used by caving enthusiasts make very good hands-free lights for oral examination and dental work (Fig. 2-8). Recently, one company released a small, waterproof light that is attached to the upper incisor plate of the speculum.[*]

Hand Floats

Perhaps more than any dental instrument, hand-held dental floats need to fit the individual practitioner (Fig. 2-9). There are several handle and grip styles, including the traditional wooden handle, hard rubber handle, foam grip, and pistol grip. Buy floats that both suit the intended purpose and fit your hand well. The various styles of hand float and their common applications are summarized in Table 2-1.

Regardless of the style of float, choose floats made of good-quality stainless steel that are sturdily constructed and have smooth edges (i.e., no sharp or rough edges that might traumatize the oral soft tissues). For floats with interchangeable blades, make sure the blade box accommodates any style of blade and has large, robust setscrews that are easily turned and resistant to wear. Some low-profile floats have interchangeable blades that are held in place with double-sided tape. The blades are easily removed by soaking the float head in acetone to loosen the tape. Floats with blades that are bonded in place should be purchased in multiples because the entire float will have to be sent to be sharpened or regritted.

Double Jeffrey gag with polyurethane wedge mouthpiece.
(Single Jeffrey gags can be ordered that come with the
strap pictured at right of each double gag with the off-
cheek hook and a polyurethane wedge mouthpiece.)

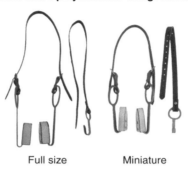

Full size   Miniature

Polyurethane wedge mouthpiece

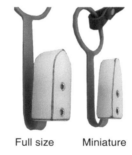

Full size   Miniature

Figure 2-6. A spool gag inserted into a horses' mouth for dental procedures should be avoided. Wedge gags are better for distributing pressure, and they are better when used in pairs. (Courtesy World Wide Equine, Inc., Glenns Ferry, Idaho.)

Float Blades

The cutting surface on equine dental float blades is made of carbide, either solid carbide or grit (carbide chips) (Fig. 2-10). The quality, or hardness, of the carbide determines the cost and longevity of the blade. The C value indicates the toughness of the carbide. Higher is better; C12 is tougher than C10, for example.

Carbide float blades are available in a range of cuts from coarse to fine. Finer blades have smaller cutting points but more points per inch, which makes the blade easier to pull and push than a coarser blade with larger (and fewer) cutting points. Finer blades also stay sharper longer. Coarse blades are used for removing large amounts of tooth material, such as when reducing waves. Medium blades remove moderate amounts of tooth, so they are more appropriate for horses that receive routine dental maintenance. Fine blades remove only small amounts of tooth material and leave a very smooth finish.

Solid carbide blades are rectangular pieces of machined carbide into which a rasp pattern has been cut. These blades are machined to be extremely sharp, but they cut in only one direction. When working on the caudal cheek teeth, the blades should be inserted into the blade box (or adhered to the float, in the case of low-profile floats) in such a way that they cut on the "pull" stroke (i.e., as the float is being pulled toward the operator) rather than on the "push" stroke. Doing so minimizes the risk of trauma to the tissues in the caudal portion of the oral cavity. When working on the more rostral teeth, it is often easier to work with the blades oriented to cut on the push stroke.

Grit blades are carbide chips bonded to a steel blank. They are less expensive than solid carbide blades. Grit blades cut in both directions (on both the push and the pull), but they require more effort to achieve the same result as a sharp solid carbide blade (Fig. 2-11).

Most solid carbide blades may be resharpened at least four times. Only the blade itself needs to be sent for sharpening, so the float can be used in the interim if a replacement blade is available. Grit blades can be regritted repeatedly, but because the carbide chips are bonded to the float blade, the entire float must be sent for regritting with most models.

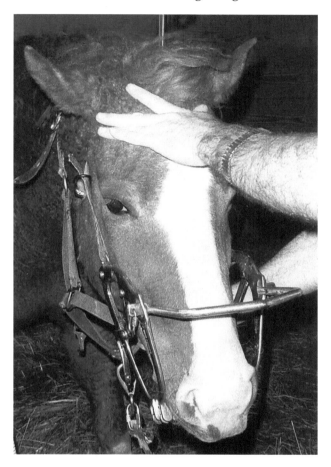

Figure 2-7. Massage the temporalis muscles for a few seconds every 10 minutes.

Extractors and Elevators

Being properly equipped for extractions makes these procedures quicker and easier, and lessens the potential for complications such as tooth breakage. Basic equipment should include a set of wolf tooth extractors (elevators and forceps), Reynolds forceps for extracting deciduous premolars (caps), and molar extractors. Use of these instruments is described in Chapters 6 and 7 (Fig. 2-12).

Wolf Tooth Extractors

Extraction of wolf teeth (the first premolar) generally is performed using wolf tooth elevators and wolf tooth forceps. Wolf tooth elevators should be of good quality; inferior quality elevators tend to blunt more easily and are more likely to break with repeated use. It is best to have at least three sizes of elevator—small, medium, and large—to accommodate the wide variability in the size of wolf teeth (Fig. 2-12).

Wolf tooth forceps should have a small head and the jaws should close tightly to firmly grip the tooth. Although one pair of forceps may do, it is best to have both straight and angled forceps. Wolf tooth forceps can also be used to extract deciduous incisors and tooth fragments.

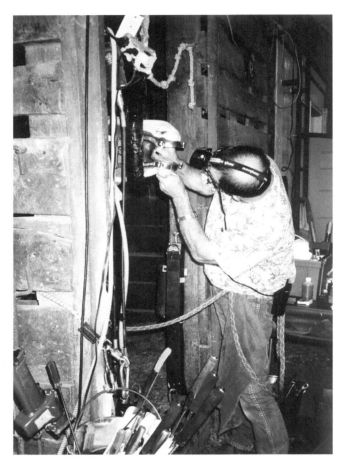

Figure 2-8. One light source with battery pack that attaches to belt.

Cap Extractors or Forceps

Reynolds-style forceps are specifically designed for extracting deciduous premolars. The handles are short and formed to fit the hand, and the head is angled, which makes one-handed extractions easier than with molar extractors. Forceps designed for the lower arcades have closed serrated heads to allow a sure grip on the more narrow lower premolar caps. Forceps designed for the upper arcades have open heads to accommodate the wider teeth (see Fig. 2-13).

Molar Extractors

Molar extractors have longer handles than cap extractors, which gives the operator more leverage when extracting permanent cheek teeth. These extractors are simple-jointed and are available with open or closed heads (Fig. 2-14). Closed-head molar extractors typically are used to extract split cheek teeth or pieces of fractured tooth. They can securely grip one half of a split tooth and even smaller tooth fragments. Open-head molar extractors are best for extracting intact molars, especially in the upper arcade (in which the teeth are wider than in the lower arcades).

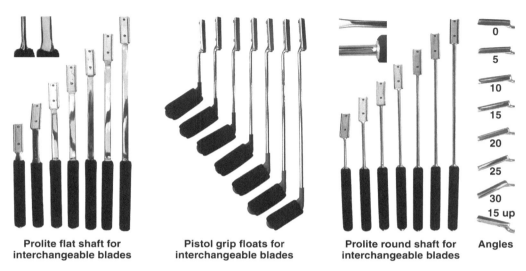

Prolite flat shaft for interchangeable blades

Pistol grip floats for interchangeable blades

Prolite round shaft for interchangeable blades

Angles

0
5
10
15
20
25
30
15 up

The above floats are all available in the head angles shown at the right. They can be used with either the solid tungsten or carbide chip blades.

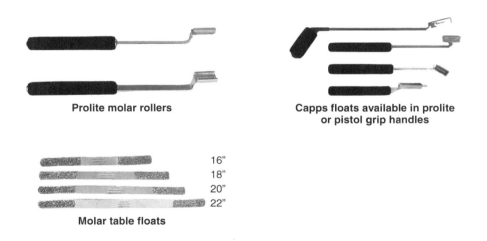

Prolite molar rollers

Capps floats available in prolite or pistol grip handles

16"
18"
20"
22"

Molar table floats

Figure 2-9. A variety of hand-held floats. (Courtesy World Wide Equine, Inc., Glenns Ferry, Idaho.)

Table 2-1	Common Uses for the Various Styles of Hand Float
Float Style	**Application**
Straight	Upper and lower cheek teeth arcades and lower caudal molars (long shaft needed)
Obtuse	Rostral upper molars; used to shape the first cheek teeth (Triadan 106 and 206) when forming bit seats; also used to remove small upper 6 hooks (see Chapter 6)
Offset	Lower arcades and lower bit seats
Upper back	Buccal cusps on the upper last two cheek teeth (this float has a very narrow, (upturned) slender head)
S-float	Finishing and for floating areas that are difficult to reach with a standard float

Detail of the Capps float head showing the three-sided tungsten carbide inserts.

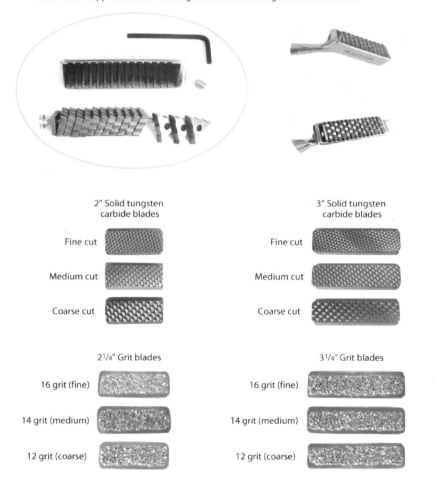

Figure 2-10. Interchangeable blades for floats. *(Courtesy World Wide Equine, Inc., Glenns Gerry, Idaho.)*

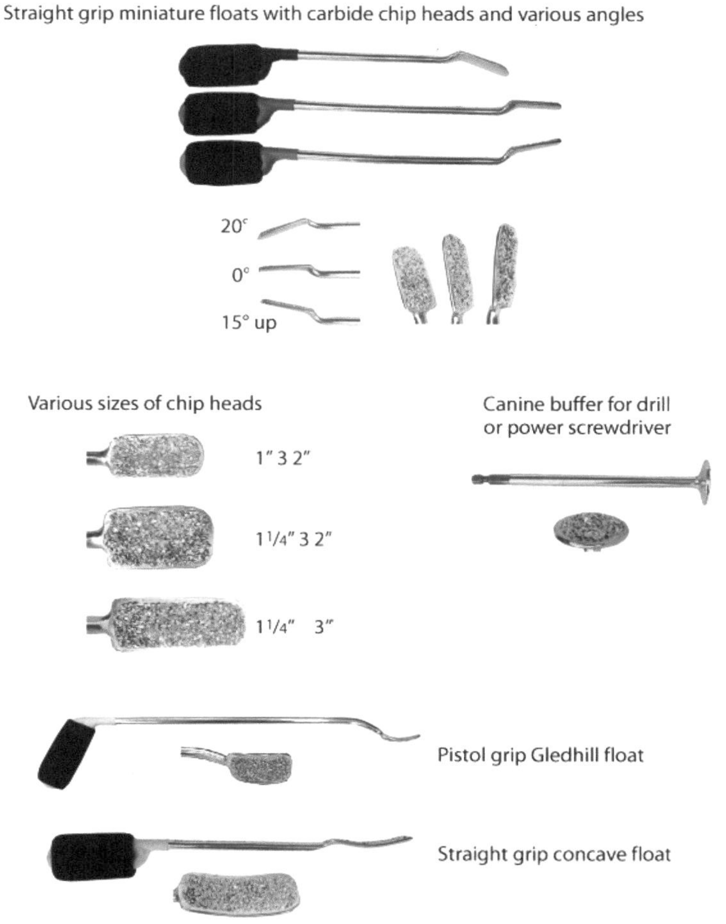

Straight grip miniature floats with carbide chip heads and various angles

20°
0°
15° up

Various sizes of chip heads

1" 3 2"

1 1/4" 3 2"

1 1/4"   3"

Canine buffer for drill or power screwdriver

Pistol grip Gledhill float

Straight grip concave float

Figure 2-11. Grit blades. (Courtesy World Wide Equine, Inc., Glenns Ferry, Idaho.)

Some molar extraction forceps are available with a built-in fulcrum. The fulcrum increases the leverage that can be applied to the tooth, making intraoral extraction of cheek teeth easier in the confines of the oral cavity (see Color Plate 56).

Molar separators or spreaders may also be needed for extraction of intact cheek teeth. Unless the tooth is already very loose, oral extractions cannot be accomplished without first loosening the tooth. Molar spreaders come in a variety of blade dimensions.

Electric Power Tools

Electric motor–driven dental instruments include motorized burrs, reciprocating floats, and rotating disks (Fig. 2-15). As with all electric equipment, care must be taken to keep the electrical connections and motor dry. In addition, a ground fault circuit interrupter (GFCI device) should always be used between the power outlet and the instrument. These devices can be found in hardware or building supply stores.

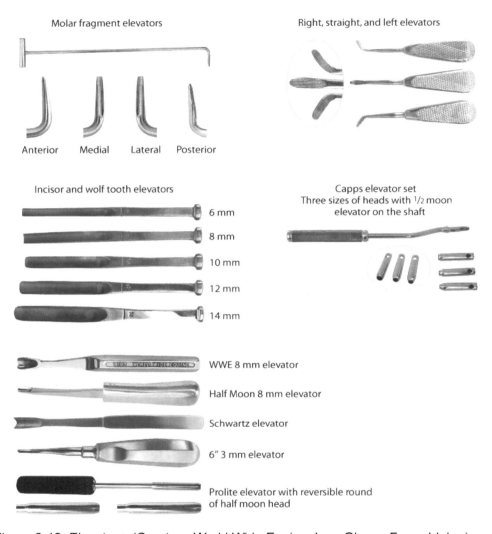

Molar fragment elevators

Anterior   Medial   Lateral   Posterior

Right, straight, and left elevators

Incisor and wolf tooth elevators

6 mm
8 mm
10 mm
12 mm
14 mm

WWE 8 mm elevator

Half Moon 8 mm elevator

Schwartz elevator

6" 3 mm elevator

Prolite elevator with reversible round
of half moon head

Capps elevator set
Three sizes of heads with 1/2 moon
elevator on the shaft

Figure 2-12. Elevators. (Courtesy World Wide Equine, Inc., Glenns Ferry, Idaho.)

Motorized Burrs

Motorized burrs are Dremel-type powered tools that are available in a range of shaft lengths, from 2 inches to 12 inches (Fig. 2-16). For these instruments to be used efficiently and safely, they should have some type of speed control, such as a foot pedal. Some motorized burrs have clutches that are designed to make them more "tissue friendly." Suction attachments are available, which can be useful for removing tooth dust and fine particles from the oral cavity during operation. Most of the currently available electric dental burrs are cable driven. These cables can break and need periodic maintenance to keep them safe.

Reciprocating Floats

Electric reciprocating floats are constructed on reciprocating saw frames. They are available in battery powered and corded models (Fig. 2-17). The stroke length ranges from 8 to 32 mm (5/16 inch to 1 1/4 inches), depending on the model. With a solid carbide blade, these floats can remove a large amount of tooth rapidly. The heavy-duty models are mostly used for wave reductions, whereas the battery-powered models are usually reserved for lighter finish work.

Extreme care should be taken when using these tools because they can damage the caudal aspect of the oral cavity. To be safe, the float head of the longer-stroke models should not be extended past the fourth cheek tooth.

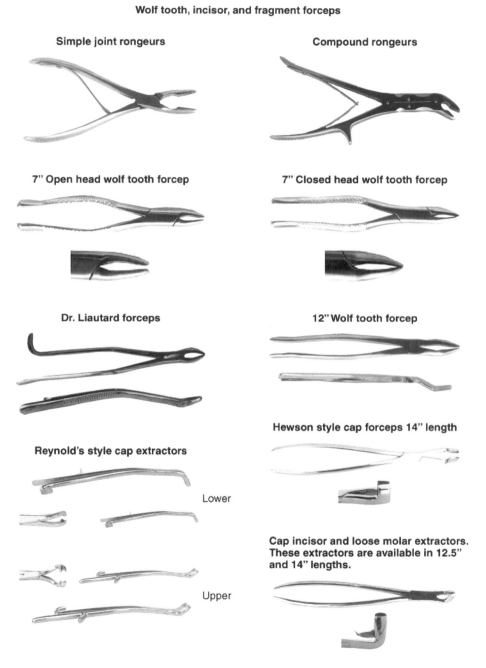

Figure 2-13. Wolf tooth extractors, wolf tooth forceps, and cap extraction forceps. (Courtesy World Wide Equine, Inc., Glenns Ferry, Idaho.)

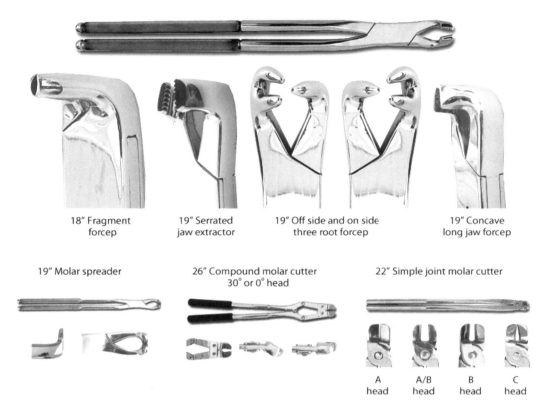

Figure 2-14. Molar extractors, spreaders, and cutters. *(Courtesy World Wide Equine, Inc., Glenns Ferry, Idaho.)*

Rotary Disks

These instruments consist of a rotating disk that is mounted on a long, sleeved shaft and powered by a variable-speed electric drill or by a motor such as a Dremel. The disk has an abrasive surface composed of carbide or industrial diamonds, depending on the coarseness desired (Figs. 2-18 and 2-19).

The PowerFloat* is a drill-powered instrument that is available only to veterinarians. Because the tungsten-carbide grinding wheel is set at 90 degrees to the shaft, this instrument can be used for any procedure that would normally be performed with a float. A solid guard surrounds the rotating disk, so this tool is very safe to use, even in the caudal reaches of the mouth (Fig. 2-20). One drawback is that the long shaft makes working on the rostral cheek teeth, canines, and incisors a little cumbersome. However, the shaft length and compact head make this tool ideal for working on the cheek teeth arcades.

The Slim Float by Eisenhut is another drill-powered disc unit, and the Horse Power Handpiece unit is now available, using a Dremel handpiece rather than a drill (all units available from World Wide Equine) (Fig. 2-21).

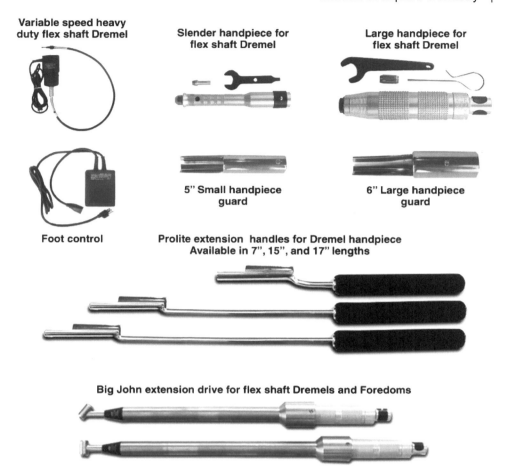

Figure 2-15. Electric power tools, motorized burrs. *(Courtesy World Wide Equine, Inc., Glenns Ferry, Idaho.)*

Pneumatic Power Tools

Pneumatic dental equipment is driven by compressed air, so an air compressor is required for operation (Fig. 2-22). With sufficient length of tubing, the air compressor can be located far enough from the work area to be barely noticeable. Thus one advantage of pneumatic instruments over electric power tools is that they are quieter. Another advantage is that pneumatic dental instruments are constructed with industrial-grade components designed to endure the mechanical fatigue of daily use.

The biggest concern with pneumatic instruments is water in the compressor. A water separator is needed to prevent water from accumulating in the compressor; both the separator and compressor tanks need to be drained daily when pneumatic equipment is used every day. If the manufacturer does not supply a water separator with the compressor, one must be added.

Another important item is an in-line oiler, which delivers constant lubrication to the instruments. In any case, it is wise to give the instruments a thorough cleaning and liberal oiling after use. Taking these few minutes periodically keeps the instruments running efficiently and extends the life of this expensive piece of equipment. As with electric dental equipment, rotary (in-line and right-angled) and reciprocating pneumatic heads are available.

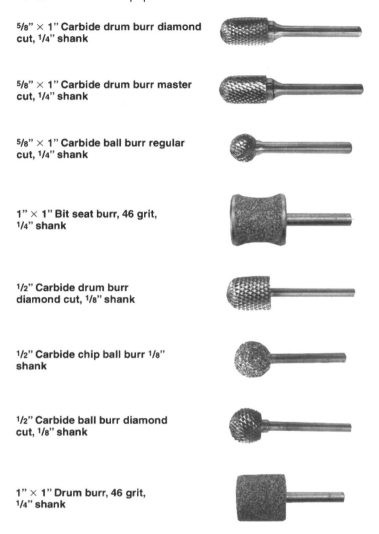

⁵/₈" × 1" **Carbide drum burr diamond cut, ¹/₄" shank**

⁵/₈" × 1" **Carbide drum burr master cut, ¹/₄" shank**

⁵/₈" × 1" **Carbide ball burr regular cut, ¹/₄" shank**

1" × 1" **Bit seat burr, 46 grit, ¹/₄" shank**

¹/₂" **Carbide drum burr diamond cut, ¹/₈" shank**

¹/₂" **Carbide chip ball burr ¹/₈" shank**

¹/₂" **Carbide ball burr diamond cut, ¹/₈" shank**

1" × 1" **Drum burr, 46 grit, ¹/₄" shank**

Figure 2-16. Assorted rotary burrs. (Courtesy World Wide Equine, Inc., Glenns Ferry, Idaho.)

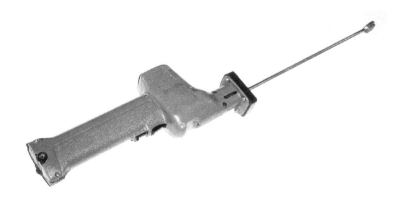

Figure 2-17. Reciprocating float.

Large head horsepower handpiece unit.
This unit includes a large dremel hand piece,
one diamond disc, one ⅛" collet, and one guard

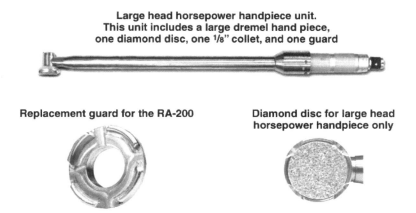

Replacement guard for the RA-200   **Diamond disc for large head**
horsepower handpiece only

Figure 2-18. RA-200 horsepower handpiece for Dremel units (13-inch shaft length, overall length of 18 inches). (Courtesy World Wide Equine, Inc., Glenns Ferry, Idaho.)

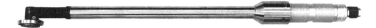

Figure 2-19. RA-250 horse power handpiece for Dremel units (13.5-inch shaft length, overall length of 18 inches). (Courtesy World Wide Equine, Inc., Glenns Ferry, Idaho.)

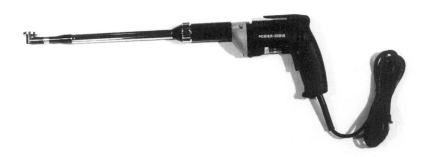

Figure 2-20. PowerFloat rotating carbide grit disc. (Courtesy D&B Equine Enterprises, Inc., Alberta, Canada.)

Rotary Burrs

Pneumatic rotary burrs may be used to remove large amounts of tooth. They have a wide range of speeds and can operate at low speeds with more torque than electric burrs, which gives the operator more control and less risk of the burr becoming "bogged down." The cutting surface of rotary burrs may be solid carbide (milled burrs), grit (chipped) carbide, or diamond coated (see Fig. 2-21).

Reciprocating Floats

Reciprocating pneumatic floats can be used for routine floating; they are used to remove large enamel points and small hooks. These floats operate with straight, angled, or specialty shafts, making them very versatile. They operate best with a solid carbide blade that is specifically designed to work with the pneumatic stroke. Pneumatic floats are very gentle on the patient and, when appropriate care is taken, they do not traumatize the caudal aspect of the oral cavity (see Fig. 2-22).

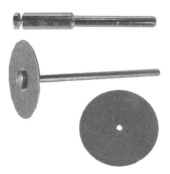

Diamond cut-off wheel with or without mandrel for cutting incisors or canines.

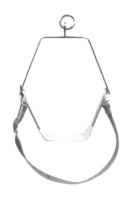

This halter is used for holding the horse's head in position. It has a leather covered foam pad to allow comfortable resting of the mandible.

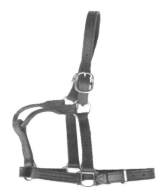

This halter has a buckle in the nose band allowing it to be easily dropped when putting on the speculum.

Figure 2-21. Rotary discs, dental frame, and dental halter. (Courtesy World Wide Equine, Inc., Glenns Ferry, Idaho.)

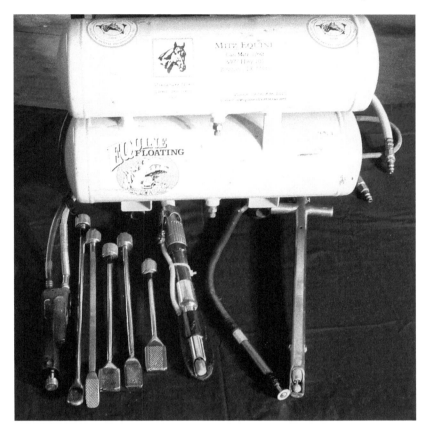

Figure 2-22. Pneumatic dental equipment by Carl Mitz. (Courtesy Tami Mitz, Brenham, TX.)

Dental Frames and Stands

A dental frame or dental halter is useful for supporting the sedated horse's head. Most dental frames are either hexagonal or circular (Fig. 2-23). Some practitioners prefer to support the horse's head using a custom-made dental stand or a modified human crutch, placed under the horse's chin. One disadvantage of this support method is that an assistant is required to keep the horse's chin on the stand and to keep the stand in place if the patient moves. Nevertheless, dental stands can come in handy when there is no overhead support from which to suspend a dental frame.

For the purpose of restraint, it is generally a good idea to keep the horse's halter on during the dentistry procedures. If the noseband cannot be expanded to comfortably accommodate the full-mouth speculum and the patient's opened mouth, the halter should be loosened and the noseband slipped off the horse's head; the poll strap can then be retightened so that the handler has some control over the horse (Fig. 2-24). Alternatively, a larger halter may be used in place of the horse's regular halter.

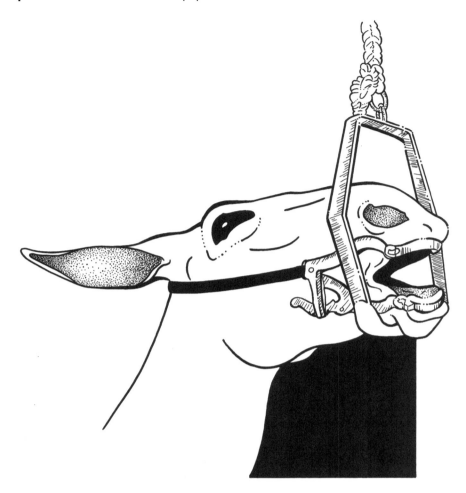

Figure 2-23. Speculum and hexagonal dental frame in use.

MOBILE EQUINE DENTISTRY CLINICS

Tom Allen

With some simple modifications, horse trailers can be customized to become mobile equine dentistry clinics (Color Plate 20). This investment is well worth considering if dentistry comprises a substantial amount of your practice activity and most of your work is done at your clients' facilities rather than your own hospital or clinic. The mobile equine dental clinic significantly increases work efficiency, because set-up and pack-up times are negligible and work conditions are consistent. The unit I currently use is a horse trailer with built-in stocks that can be modified to accommodate any size horse from a miniature horse to a draft horse. With a loading ramp that is 6 feet long and an interior height of 8 feet, I encounter very few problems loading horses into the stocks (Color Plate 21 and 22).

Equipment for Small Patients

Dentistry on small ponies, donkeys, and miniature breeds (horses, mules, and donkeys) can be a challenge, because few manufacturers make instruments designed for use in small equids. However, that situation is changing (Figs. 2-25 to 2-27). Smaller specula are now available; stocks can be custom-made for small patients; and some of the newer hand floats with short shafts and slender blades developed for specific uses in full-size horses are well suited for use in small patients. As the demand increases, veterinarians will likely see an increase in the availability and range of instruments designed specifically for use in small equine patients. (Dental procedures in miniature horses are described in Chapter 8.)

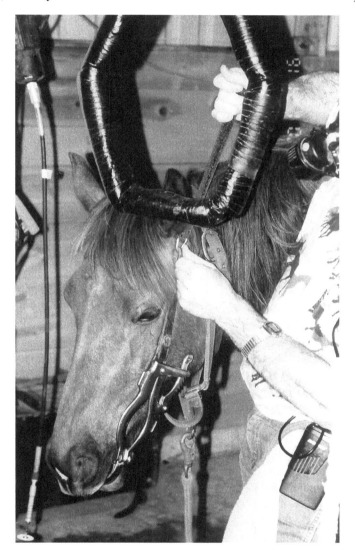

Figure 2-24. The halter is used around the sedated patient's neck. (Courtesy Angel Hope, Harrison, AR.)

EQUIPMENT MAINTENANCE

Carl Mitz and Tom Allen

Regular maintenance is necessary to keep dental instruments clean and functioning efficiently. Maintenance can simply involve cleaning for hand floats or complete breakdown and servicing for power equipment. Frequent dismantling and cleaning of all equipment is recommended by the suppliers.

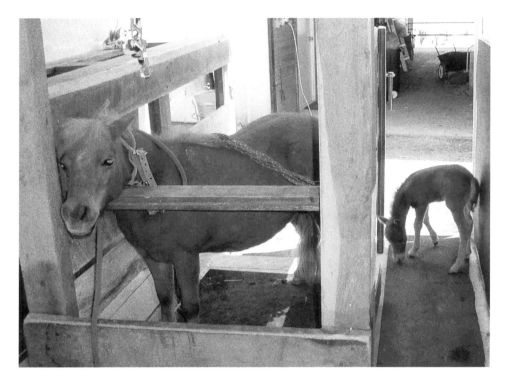

Figure 2-25. A miniature horse in place in my "horse dental chair."

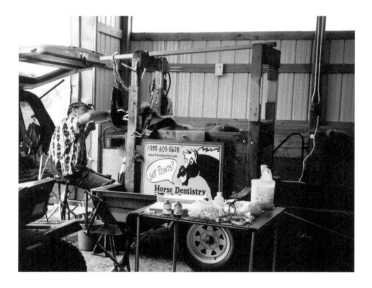

Figure 2-26. Stocks for miniatures on a small utility trailer.

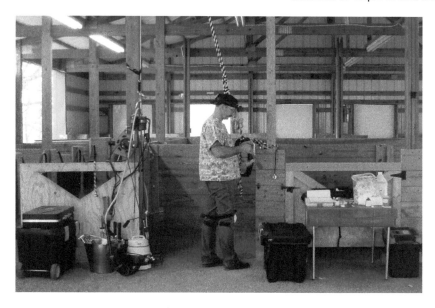

Figure 2-27. Knee pads are important if the patient is not elevated.

Hand Instruments

Many dental practitioners routinely soak their instruments in dilute chlorhexidine solution before use, between patients, and even during a procedure (when that instrument is not being used). Plastic separator tubes are available to prevent the carbide blades from knocking against one other and being blunted while in the work bucket (Color Plate 23).

After each appointment, thoroughly clean the blades of the hand floats to remove any tooth material, food debris, blood, and other tissue. Remove the blade and clean the blade box before replacing the blade and tightening the setscrews. At this time, check the sharpness of the blade. Also inspect the shafts of the floats for defects or burrs that might cause injury to the patient or to you. If dental elevators or extractors have been used, also clean them thoroughly.

Power Instruments

Rotary burrs should be cleaned of all debris daily. Lubrication is very important for the longevity of these instruments; without lubrication, water will rust the bearings in the handpieces, causing them to seize. So, periodically lubricate the cable shaft that drives the handpiece on electric burrs. A few drops of oil can save a lot of time and money. With any power instrument, be sure to follow all recommendations made by the manufacturer for maintenance and servicing.

*Wearing Bros. suspension bar, World Wide Equine, Inc., Glenns Ferry, ID 83623.

*Lochner speculum, Equi-Dent Technologies, Inc., PO Box 5877, Sparks, NV 89432.

*SpecBiteLite, Equine Dental Instruments, Reno, NV 89506.

*D & B Equine Enterprises, Inc., 207 Silverhill Way NW, Calgary, Alberta, Canada T3B 4K9.

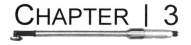

CHAPTER 3

Safety Issues and Restraint Procedures

Tom Allen, Tom Johnson, Richard O. Miller

SAFETY ISSUES

Patient Safety

Patient safety is an important consideration whenever working with a horse. For dental procedures, patient safety should be considered from the time the practitioner first approaches the horse to the point at which the horse is returned to its normal environment and state of awareness (i.e., until any sedation has worn off or has been reversed). In addition to the animal welfare aspect, taking steps to ensure patient safety is important to avoid loss of client confidence and legal action should the horse be harmed while under the practitioner's care.

When working at the client's facility, it is often best to perform routine dental work in the horse's stall (Color Plate 24). Before beginning any work, inspect the stall for any items that could cause injury to the horse, the assistant-handler, or you, such as protruding nails, screws, or splinters. If these items cannot be removed, another stall should be used.

Sedation, although making the practitioner's job easier and lessening the horse's reaction to manipulations, can add a degree of complexity because it interferes with the patient's coordination. Thus it is important to place the horse in surroundings that minimize the chance of injury before administering a sedative or beginning any dental procedures. Chemical restraint is discussed at the end of this chapter.

Footing

Whether or not the horse is sedated, it is important that any procedures be conducted in an area with nonslip footing, such as wood shavings or sawdust, dirt, gravel, sand, rubber matting, or rubber bricks, particularly if the horse is shod (Color Plate 25). Surfaces such as bare concrete, clay brick, and wood are unsafe, especially when wet. Areas with such surfaces should not be used for any procedure to which the horse might react evasively, particularly if the horse is sedated. In fact, sedated horses probably should not even be walked across such surfaces. When performing dental procedures in a stall, footing usually is not a problem, because most stalls are bedded with materials that minimize slipping.

Human Safety

Ensuring the safety of the patient also contributes to the safety of the humans in attendance. Adequate patient restraint is another key factor in ensuring the safety of the operator and assistants, including any person holding the horse. The horse is the most unpredictable element in the equation and the one most likely to injure the operator, assistant, or handler.

Although sedation generally decreases the risk of injury to the operator and assistants, it is important to remember that horses sedated with xylazine and related drugs (e.g., detomidine) may kick out suddenly and with surprising force and accuracy if handled around the hindquarters. I have observed this dangerous reaction in perhaps 1 in 1000 horses on which I have performed dental procedures, none of them "known kickers." So, when using these sedatives, do not allow anyone to stand or walk behind the horse in the "strike zone" while the patient is sedated (Color Plate 26). Chemical restraint is discussed further at the end of the chapter.

One other safety item worth mentioning is a chest strap: a strong leather or nylon strap that can be used to prevent the horse from pushing forward when dental work is being performed in the doorway of a stall. One option is to use a girth strap with short chains attached to each end (Color Plate 27). When the occasion demands, the strap is attached across the stall doorway to prevent the horse from pushing forward (which sometimes happens in horses sedated with butorphanol). This strap is also a useful safety device when performing dental extractions on a standing horse (see Chapter 7). The strap protects the operator if the horse suddenly launches itself forward and upward during the procedure.

Liability Issues

While a practitioner is examining and treating a horse, that animal is the responsibility of the practitioner. To minimize injury to any other person, and thus limit legal liability, it is important to determine the competence of any person who will be near or handling the horse. Children and any person who is physically or mentally impaired should not be permitted to remain in the work area. If you have any doubt about the ability of the owner or agent to restrain the horse, make other arrangements (e.g., have someone else hold the horse, or rely on sedation and a dental frame alone to restrain the horse).

Allowing the owner or trainer to look in or palpate the horse's mouth can be a good educational and public relations exercise (Color Plate 28). However, that person's safety is paramount. Make sure the horse is adequately restrained and is unable to bite down on the person's hand or swing its head and thus injure the person's arm. Before allowing the owner or trainer to put a hand inside the horse's mouth, check that the speculum is secure. Also be sure to give adequate instructions on how to palpate the oral structures safely. It is not a good idea to allow an owner or trainer to handle any power equipment.

It is also important to forewarn the handler to stay clear of the horse's head when the horse is wearing a full-mouth speculum. If the horse swings its head suddenly, any person standing within range may be injured by the speculum. Use of sedation minimizes, but does not eliminate, the risk of this type of injury.

Work-Related Injuries

Even when using power equipment, dental procedures can be physically demanding on the operator. To minimize work-related strain and injury, it is important to develop efficient work habits and ease the load on your body wherever possible. Some procedures can be performed while seated on a lightweight, collapsible stool (e.g., a campstool), which reduces back strain (Fig. 3-1). However, the horse must be well sedated and adequately restrained if dental procedures are to be performed by an operator seated in front of the horse. I found that as I became more efficient, I no longer needed to use the stool.

FACILITIES

Working at the Client's Facility

When asked to perform routine dental procedures at the client's facility (whether the client's own property or a boarding facility), it is important that suitable shelter be available. The sheltered area should, at the very least, provide protection from rain (particularly important when using motorized equipment) and should be dark enough to allow good visualization of the oral cavity using a portable light source. Bright sunlight makes thorough visualization of the horse's oral cavity very difficult and can be a strain on the examiner's eyes.

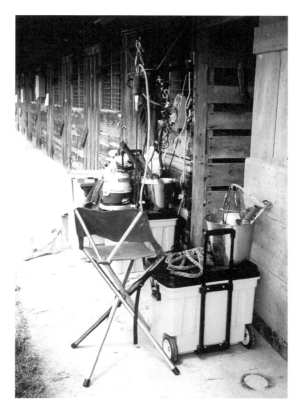

Figure 3-1. A lightweight campstool can be useful at times.

A second requirement is a supply of clean water. If using electrically powered dental equipment or light sources, it is also necessary to have a reliable electricity supply. In addition, a GFCI should be used between the electricity source and the motorized equipment (i.e., between the power outlet and the patient). These devices can be found in hardware or building supply stores, and are plugged into the electric outlet. They should be tested before each use to make sure they are functioning properly. If they do not "trip" when the test button is pushed, they will not break the circuit when voltage to ground is present and are not safe to use. When functioning properly, GFCI devices will break the circuit before the patient or practitioner can be harmed by stray voltage.

It is highly desirable when using a dental frame to have a strong beam from which to suspend the dental frame and thus support the patient's head. When performing dental work in a stall, the dental frame can be suspended from the framing above the stall door; a sturdy rafter may also be used (Fig. 3-2). Before I started using my customized horse trailer for all dental work (see Chapter 2), I carried ropes for this purpose in my truck, and some large screw eyes and a battery-powered drill so that I could suspend the dental frame in various locations, depending on the stall construction.

Because routine dental procedures rarely are performed on an emergency basis, it is the practitioner's prerogative to refuse to perform dental procedures in unsuitable facilities. Experience has taught me that performing dentistry in less-than-ideal surroundings can be difficult, time-consuming, stressful, and even unsafe. I have refused to perform routine dentistry at facilities that do not meet the basic standards of suitability described earlier.

Practitioners who are persuaded to work in substandard or unsafe conditions perform less efficiently, do lower quality work with less enjoyment and more risk, and rob patients of the full benefits of thorough dental care. Make your requirements for shelter, electricity, and water clear to clients before the first appointment is made; very few equine facilities do not have these items. If you insist upon having decent facilities in which to work, the client will find a way to provide them. For example, the client may choose to transport the horse to a friend's barn or the trainer's facility. Some clients have built an appropriate work area on their property, on being told what is required. Such an area can also be used for other veterinary procedures and for farriery care.

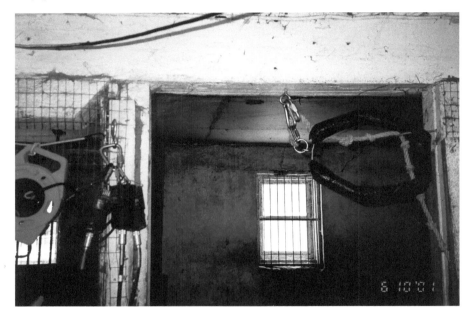

Figure 3-2. A dental frame is suspended from a strong beam. Even a 2 x 4 will support the horse's head during dental procedures.

Working at Your Own Facility

If you have your own facility, whether a hospital or simply a barn, a chute or stocks can be used very effectively if equipped to accommodate the way you work (Color Plate 29). Exact specifications for design of equine stocks may be found elsewhere. Generally, stocks work well for the average-size horse if their interior dimensions are approximately 76 cm (30 inches) wide and 2m (6½ feet) long. If the flooring of the stocks area is concrete, it should be covered with rubber matting or painted with a nonslip material.

Modifications to basic metal equine stocks for dental work should include an overhead device from which to suspend the dental frame used to support the horse's head. Although various configurations may be used, all that is needed is a bar, positioned well above the horse's head, which protrudes approximately 90 cm (3 feet) forward of the chest barrier. A rope attached to the dental frame is run over the bar and tied such that the horse's head is supported at a comfortable height for both the horse and the operator.

The stocks can also be adapted to create a place from which to suspend routinely used items of equipment at work level. For example, a horizontal support can be extended approximately 90 cm (3 feet) forward of the chest barrier and the instruments suspended from this bar. Such adaptations can add considerably to your comfort and efficiency when performing dental procedures.

RESTRAINT

The following are the three basic types of restraint, and each has a place in equine dentistry:
1. Behavioral—response to voice commands or the handler's position or movement
2. Physical—halter, stocks or chute, skin twitch, twitch, lip chain
3. Chemical—sedatives and analgesics, regional anesthesia
Although a well-behaved horse may require only behavioral and light physical restraint,

chemical restraint is often necessary in nervous or frightened horses. An argument could be made for the importance of training horses to tolerate routine dental procedures; however, in most circumstances the practitioner has little time to devote to training or desensitizing horses to dental manipulations. Thus it is often better to use chemical restraint sooner rather than later in anxious or uncooperative patients. For safety reasons I consider chemical restraint to be a necessity when using power equipment to perform dental procedures.

A lip twitch is commonly used by some practitioners to restrain uncooperative horses for dental procedures. However, a few horses react violently to the twitch, striking out suddenly. Because dental procedures necessitate standing in front of the horse, the dental operator is in a very dangerous position should a horse react so to the twitch. Considering the availability, cost, variety, and safety of currently available sedatives, I believe that using a twitch to restrain a horse for dental work is unnecessarily risky.

Routine Chemical Restraint

α-2 Agonists

Deep sedation is required for most dental work that is performed using motorized equipment. My preference for sedation is a mixture of xylazine and detomidine. I use a 3:2:1 mixture (by volume) of xylazine:detomidine:butorphanol tartrate. This combination is administered intravenously (IV) at an initial dosage of 2.5 to 3ml per 1000 pounds of body weight. Most light breed horses (those weighing between 800 and 1200 pounds) receive this amount. Smaller patients tend to require more sedative per pound of body weight. For example, miniature horses weighing 100 to 300 pounds typically receive 0.75 to 1.25ml of a 10:1 xylazine: detomidine (by volume) mixture. Large horses tend to require less sedative per pound of body weight. For example, draft breeds receive the same initial dose as light breed horses.

The initial dose is adequate for oral examination and dental charting in most patients. However, I often need to give additional sedative before performing any corrective procedures. The amount of sedative given at this point and subsequently during the procedure is highly variable; I usually give the combination in increments of 1.5 to 2ml. Depending on the patient and on the length of the procedure, the total cumulative dose of the xylazine-detomidine mixture may be as much as 5 ml, although that amount is unusual. Having experienced several "claustrophobic" reactions in patients, I have recently increased the amount of detomidine used in horses. I administer it before the patient nears the trailer I now use for all my work.

Some breeds, such as Missouri foxtrotters and Tennessee walking horses, require much smaller amounts of sedative than expected for their size. It is not unusual for these horses to receive a total cumulative dose of only 2.5ml of the xylazine-detomidine mixture for the entire procedure (oral examination and dental work). All cases must be evaluated on an individual basis; sedation should be adequate to prevent excitement reactions.

Reversal of α-2 Agonists

The sedative effects of α-2 agonists such as xylazine and detomidine can be reversed by administration of yohimbine or tolazoline. I routinely use a reversal agent after completing the dental procedure and in instances in which the patient is excessively sedated (e.g., the horse is in danger of falling or lying down or is too uncoordinated for safety). I recommend drawing up an appropriate dose of the reversal agent before injecting the sedative, just in case the horse responds unexpectedly to the dose of sedative given and becomes overly sedated.

The reversal agent I use with the xylazine-detomidine combination described earlier is yohimbine. I give 30 to 60mg (3 to 6ml of 10mg/ml yohimbine solution) IV, depending on the amount of sedative given and on how deeply sedated the horse appears. Typically, horses are alert and coordinated within 5 minutes of receiving the yohimbine. (NOTE: There have been cases of unexplained death in horses associated with administration of a methylcellulose-based yohimbine product. For this reason I only use aqueous formulations of yohimbine.) Yohimbine injections must be given very slowly!

Butorphanol

If the patient is deeply sedated yet still too uncooperative for dental procedures to be performed safely and efficiently, I administer butorphanol (Torbugesic*) at an average dose of 5mg IV (0.5ml of 10mg/ml solution) per horse. Higher doses of butorphanol cause some horses to become "pushy" (i.e., the horse seems impelled to walk forward). In this situation the chest strap described on p. 44 is invaluable when working in a stall; when using stocks or a chute, the chest bar effectively prevents the horse from moving forward.

An added benefit to administering butorphanol for dental work is that it tends to "quiet" the horse's tongue. Movement of the horse's tongue can impede some dental procedures, such as shaping a bit seat on the first cheek teeth (see Chapter 6).

Valium

In patients that persistently shake their heads despite adequate sedation, I often administer diazepam (Valium†) at a dose of 2.5 to 10mg IV (0.5 to 2ml of 5mg/ml solution) per horse. Some patients become mildly ataxic for a short period, so be sure the patient is in a safe area before administering diazepam.

In rare instances, no combination or amount of sedatives, analgesics, or muscle relaxants is adequate to ensure the patient's cooperation. In these horses it is a struggle to do a thorough dental examination and perform corrective procedures. Fortunately, this situation is extremely uncommon.

Recordkeeping

All medications given (sedatives, analgesics, and reversal agents) should be noted in the medical record or on the dental chart, including amount(s) and time(s) administered. This practice avoids items being missed when the fee is calculated at the end of the procedure. In addition, the record serves as a useful reminder of how the horse responded to sedation for the next time you work on that patient (Color Plate 30). Be sure to comply with federal regulations concerning the storage, use, and reporting of "scheduled" drugs such as butorphanol, morphine, and diazepam.

Chemical Restraint for Major Extractions

Some dental extractions can be performed via the oral cavity in the standing, sedated horse (see Chapter 7) (Color Plate 31). The combination of sedative and analgesic agents I prefer for extractions in standing horses is the xylazine:detomidine:butorphanol mixture discussed earlier, followed by morphine at a dosage of 150 to 300mg (10 to 20ml of 15 mg/ml solution) per 1000 pounds of body weight, by slow IV injection. The morphine is administered after adequate sedation has been achieved with the xylazine-detomidine combination. In some patients it is necessary to repeat xylazine-detomidine administration during the procedure.

The effects of the xylazine-detomidine combination are reversed with yohimbine following the procedure. I also routinely reverse the effects of morphine by administering naloxone at a dose of 2mg IV for the average horse. I have observed that when morphine is not reversed, the horse may be inappetant and restless for the next 24 to 36 hours. When naloxone is administered, most horses are alert within 5 to 10 minutes, and they eat well and otherwise behave normally following the procedure.

Butorphanol tartrate may also be used as an effective analgesic for extraction of teeth, and may be reversed with naloxone also.

Some dental practitioners use regional anesthesia (nerve blocks) for standing extractions. I have not needed to use regional anesthesia for molar extractions. I have, however, infused local anesthetic agents around the tooth for some wolf tooth extractions and removal of deciduous incisors (see Chapter 6). If I cannot perform the extraction using the sedative-analgesic combination described earlier, I recommend extraction under general anesthesia at a surgical facility.

*SmithKline Beecham, Exton, Pa.

†Miles Inc., Shawnee Mission, Kan.

*Fort Dodge Animal Health, Fort Dodge, Iowa.

†Elkins-Sinn, Cherry Hill, NJ.

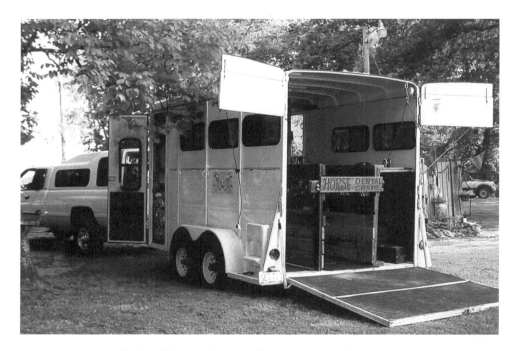

Color Plate 1. My mobile equine dentistry unit.

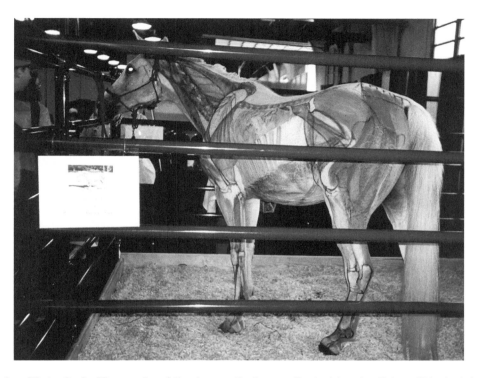

Color Plate 2. A, The parts of the horse that are affected by dentistry. (*Photo taken at Equitana in Louisville, Kentucky, June 1998.*)

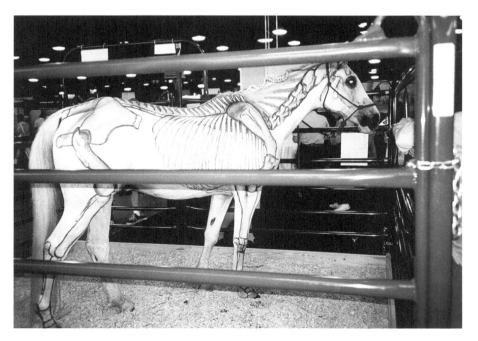

Color Plate 2. B, The parts of the horse that are affected by dentistry. (*Photo taken at Equitana in Louisville, Kentucky, June 1998.*)

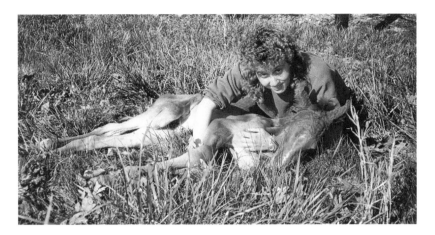

Color Plate 3. Helping their horses live longer is a valuable service to your clients.

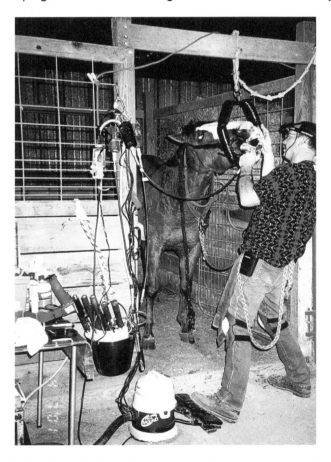

Color Plate 4. More than just two floats and a bucket.

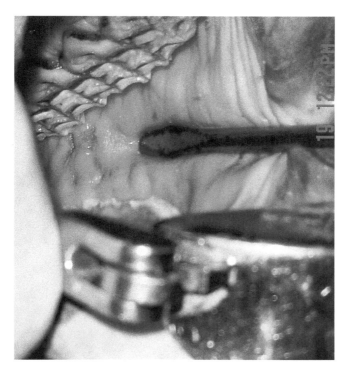

Color Plate 5. Buccal ulcerations from sharp points. (*Courtesy Joe Allen, Edinboro, PA.*)

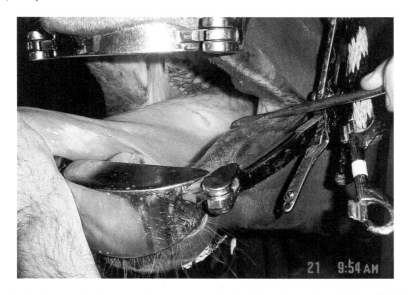

Color Plate 6. Lacerated tongue from sharp teeth. (*Courtesy Joe Allen, Edinboro, PA.*)

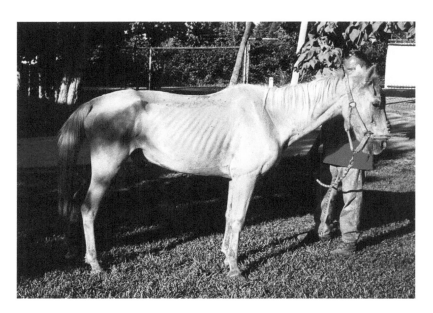

Color Plate 7. A, 19-year-old gelding before thorough dentistry.

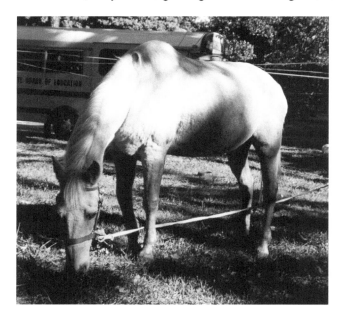

Color Plate 7. B, After thorough dentistry, 3 months later.

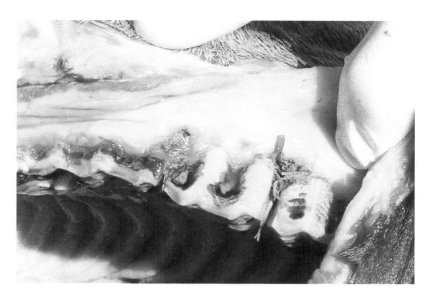

Color Plate 8. Periodontal disease in a cadaver. (*Photo taken at the International Association of Equine Dentistry [IAED] convention, Ocala, Florida, 2002. Courtesy Tami Mitz, Brenham, TX.*)

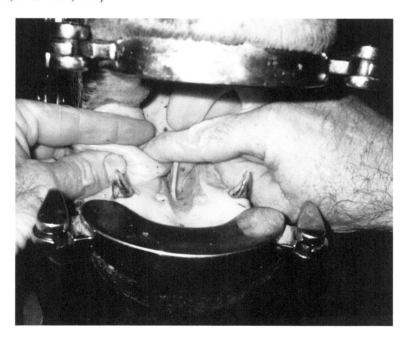

Color Plate 9. Sharp Canines.

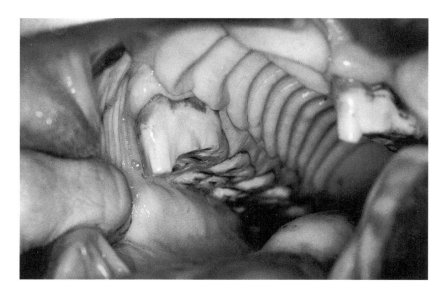

Color Plate 10. Upper 6 hooks.

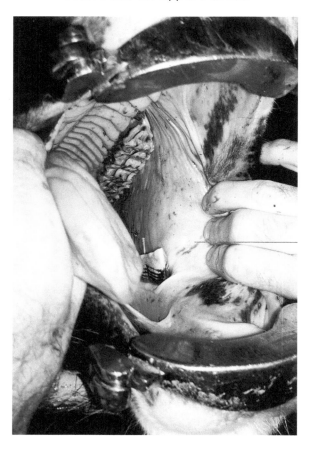

Color Plate 11. Lower 6 ramps.

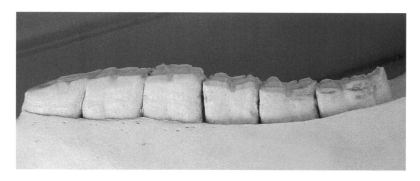

Color Plate 12. Waves, lower 11 ramps.

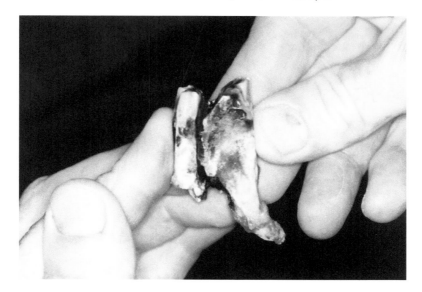

Color Plate 13. Sagittally fractured upper 9s.

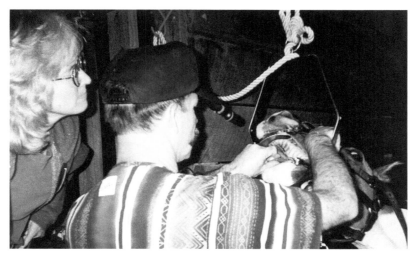

Color Plate 14. Pointing out dental problems to a horse's owner.

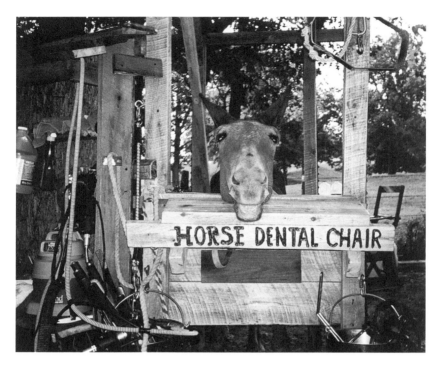

Color Plate 15. A, The front of one of my reminder cards.

YOUR HORSE IS DUE FOR
ROUTINE DENTAL MAINTENANCE!

6 month:_____

yearly:_____

OR:_____

Call or email for an appointment!

email: **tallen @horsedentist .com**

phone: **1-888-603-5628**

website: **www. horsedentist .com**

**Dr. Allen is often booked 4 to 6
weeks in advance.**

Schedule your appointment ahead!

JOIN OUR LIST MEMBERS

by visiting our website & follow
the steps to register. You will receive a

MONTHLY SCHEDULING UPDATE

for making appointments in advance.

Tom Allen DVM I.A.E.D./C
Dr. Allen's Horse Dentistry

Route 1 Box 176E
Patterson, MO 63956

Color Plate 15. B, The back of one of my reminder cards. (*Copyright 1999, Dawn
Sperry-Allen.*)

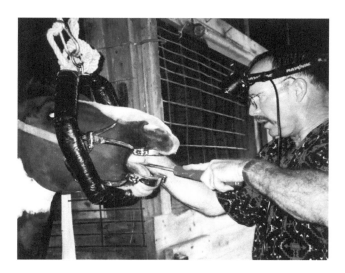

Color Plate 16. Dr. Allen using a hand float. This horse is sedated, with head supported, facilitating visualization of work, but making hand work more difficult.

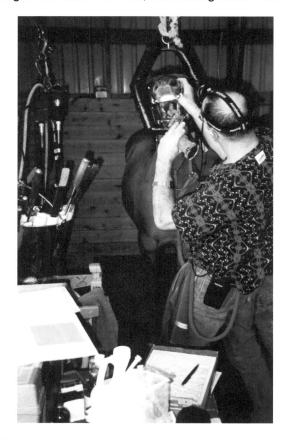

Color Plate 17. Extensive equipment must be set up within reach for power dentistry. Sedation of the patient decreases the chance of disruption from a forward lunge. A bar or strap in front of the patient is a good idea too. (*Courtesy Angel Hope, Harrison, AR.*)

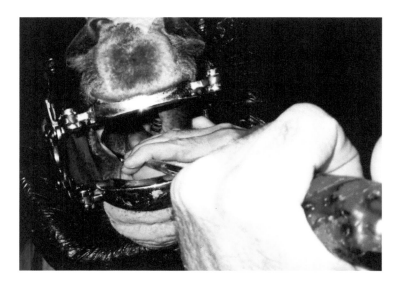

Color Plate 18. Master hand tools first.

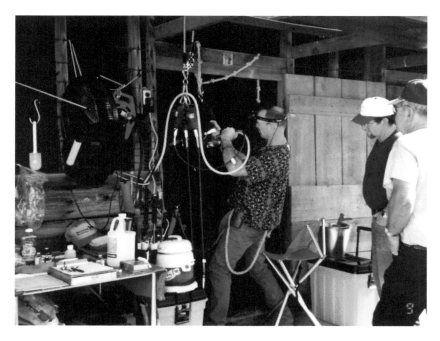

Color Plate 19. One set-up with power equipment and hand floats. Note skull under the table for demonstration of points to owners.

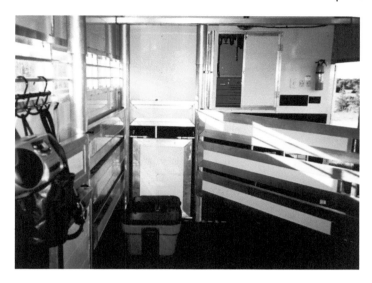

Color Plate 20. A mobile dentistry unit. (*Courtesy Dr. Tom Johnson, Grass Lake, MI.*)

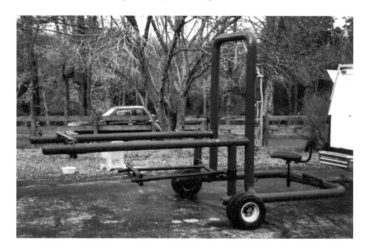

Color Plate 21. Mobile stocks. (*Courtesy Dr. John Haffner, Columbus, TN.*)

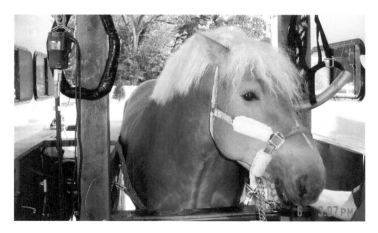

Color Plate 22. A patient in place in my "horse dental chair."

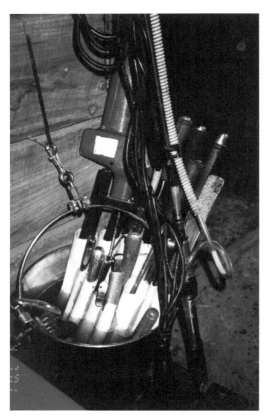

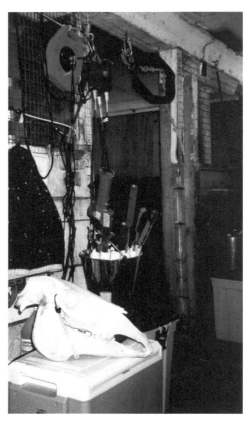

Color Plate 23. Plastic separator tubes plus a wooden disc at the bottom of disinfectant bucket prolong the lives of float blades.

Color Plate 24. Many dental practitioners set up their equipment in front of a stall.

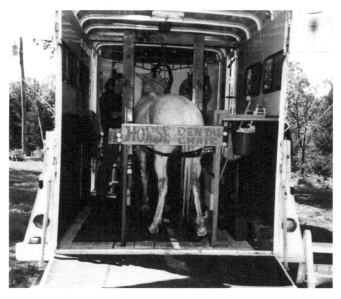

Color Plate 25. Rubber matting on wood or concrete provides secure footing. (*Courtesy Michelle Hutto, Bonne Terre, MO.*)

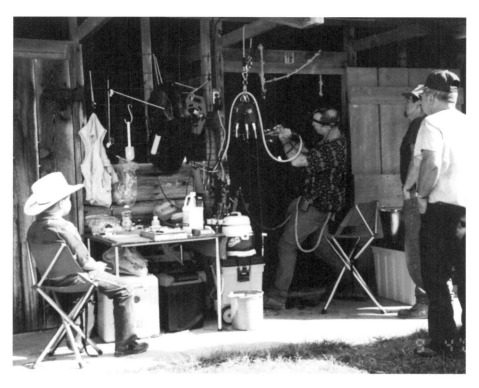

Color Plate 26. When using a stall, the patient can still leave abruptly, so keep observers at a distance, except for brief periods during examination.

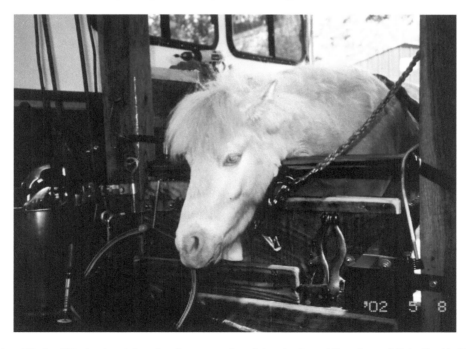

Color Plate 27. A chest barrier is a good safety device. (*Courtesy Michelle Hutto, Bonne Terre, MO.*)

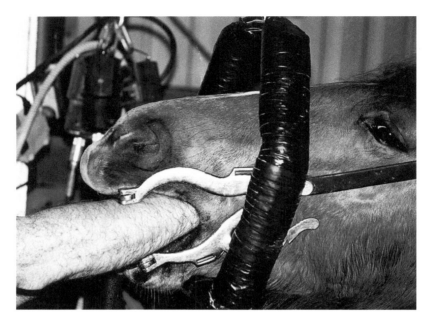

Color Plate 28. A, After the practitioner examines the horse, **B** [below], the client may be very impressed by palpating the same features.

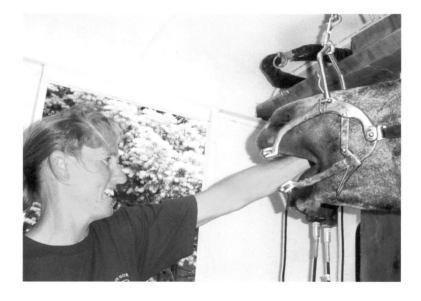

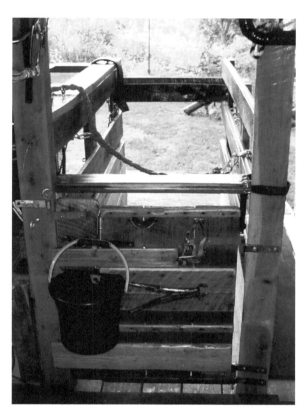

Color Plate 29. A set of stocks can make your work much more efficient. This one is in my mobile dental unit. (*The old speculum and molar cutter parts are decoration.*)

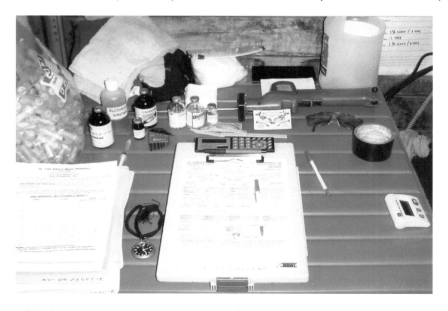

Color Plate 30. A table set-up is within reach of the practitioner, adjacent to the work area. (*Courtesy Joe Allen, Edinboro, PA.*)

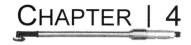

CHAPTER 4

Examination

Tom Allen

PHYSICAL EXAMINATION

Evaluation of the dental patient should begin with a brief physical examination. As I approach the horse, or as the horse is led toward me, I note the way the horse moves, its general body condition, and its demeanor. Body condition is recorded on the dental chart (see Fig. 1-7). The body condition scoring system, which grades body condition on a scale from 1 (emaciated) to 9 (obese), can be used. I use a simplified system, grading the horse's body condition as overweight, good, ribby, or emaciated. Most of the horses I see in my equine dentistry practice fit into the first two categories.

I then perform a basic physical examination, recording resting heart rate, respiratory rate, and other findings on the dental chart or medical record. (NOTE: These indices should be evaluated before the horse is sedated.) Any apparent cause for abnormal values (e.g., excitement or apprehension causing an elevation in heart rate) should be noted. Next, I observe and palpate the face and head for asymmetry, noting any abnormal findings on the record. In particular, I palpate both TMJs, maxillae, and mandibles. In my experience, asymmetry of the TMJs is a common finding (the majority of horses have a more prominent right TMJ than left); eruption cysts (bony swellings overlying the roots of unerupted cheek teeth) are also common findings (Fig. 4-1).

It is also worthwhile inquiring of the owner or caretaker (e.g., trainer, rider) whether the horse has been exhibiting any behavioral abnormalities associated with eating or with riding or driving. Briefly note any such observations in the record. Any report of lameness should also be regarded as potentially important information. Horses with long ramps on the lower 11s (see Chapter 5) may exhibit an apparent hind limb lameness when ridden that is probably associated with pressure on the tissues immediately behind the upper 11s. Removing these ramps often resolves the lameness.

ORAL EXAMINATION WITHOUT A SPECULUM

Examination of the oral cavity is best performed with the aid of a full-mouth speculum and light source. The caudal part of the oral cavity and the cheek teeth arcades in the conscious horse *cannot* be thoroughly examined any other way. However, there are some aspects of dental structure and function that are best evaluated before the speculum is applied (Fig. 4-2), including the following:
- Rostral-caudal movement of the mandible
- Incisor structure and position
- Incisor line
- Incisor table angle
- Molar occlusion

Before examining the horse's mouth, I usually sedate the horse, as described in Chapter 3.

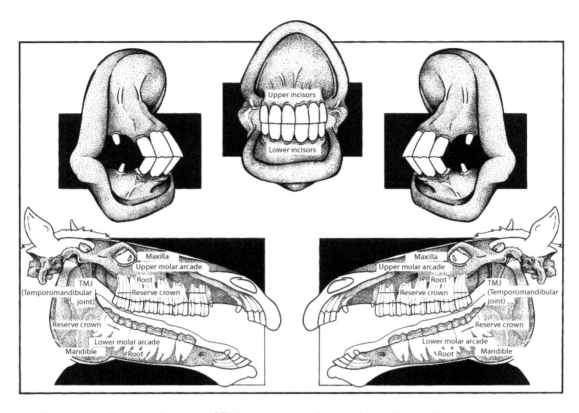

Figure 4-1. The relationship of TMJ to the arcades; incisor views without speculum.

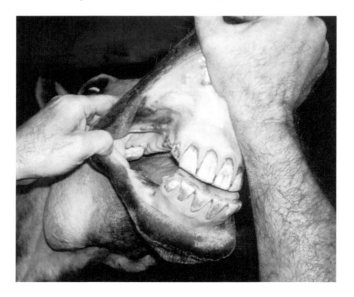

Figure 4-2. Examine the incisors before placing the speculum.

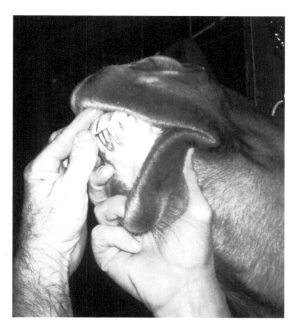

Figure 4-3. Determining the anterior-posterior (rostral-caudal) movement.

Rostral-Caudal Movement of the Mandible

In a normal horse, the TMJs allow a small amount of rostral and caudal movement of the mandibles in relation to the maxillae as the horse flexes and extends its poll or during mastication. Rostral-caudal movement of the mandible can be evaluated simply by noting the relationship between the upper and lower incisor arcades at different head positions.

Once the horse is sedated and its head drops, gently part the horse's lips and note the position of the rostral (labial) margin of the central lower incisors relative to that of the upper incisors. Then raise the horse's head and extend the poll (i.e., lift the horse's chin) as much as possible without using excessive force, and note the position of the lower incisors relative to the uppers; the lower incisors should have slid caudally several millimeters. Record the amount of rostral-caudal excursion on the dental chart (Figs. 4-3 to 4-5).

It is normal for horses to have 6 to 8 mm (approx. $1/4$ inch) of rostral-caudal excursion when assessed in this manner. If the horse's head is raised to a greater height or the poll is extended further, greater excursion may be noted. Horses with severe hooks, ramps, steps, waves, or excessive transverse ridges involving the cheek teeth (see Chapter 5) often have little or no rostral-caudal excursion until the dental abnormality is corrected. In many cases the client notices an immediate improvement in the horse's behavior or performance once the rostral-caudal range of movement is restored by proper dental treatment.

Incisors

After evaluating and recording the amount of rostral-caudal excursion, I place the patient's chin in the dental frame. I then part the horse's lips and inspect the incisors (Color Plate 32), noting the nature and position or orientation of any abnormalities on the dental chart. Common findings include missing incisors, wedge (slant) mouth, loose or damaged deciduous incisors (caps), and damaged permanent incisors. Less common abnormalities include supernumerary (extra) incisors, displaced incisors, underjet or overjet, and underbite ("hog" or "sow" mouth) or overbite ("parrot mouth"). These abnormalities are described and illustrated in Chapter 5.

Incisor Line

When viewed from in front of the horse, the line where the upper and lower incisor tables meet (the incisor line) should be horizontal. Abnormal findings include wedge mouth, smile, and frown. In wedge mouth (also called *slant* or *diagonal mouth*), the incisor line deviates from horizontal by a few degrees (i.e., the line is straight but slopes from one side of the mouth to the other). A smile denotes ventral curvature (the line dips in the center of the incisor arcade, being higher at the corners than at the center). A frown denotes dorsal curvature (the line is higher in the center than at the corners). The significance of these abnormalities is discussed in Chapter 5.

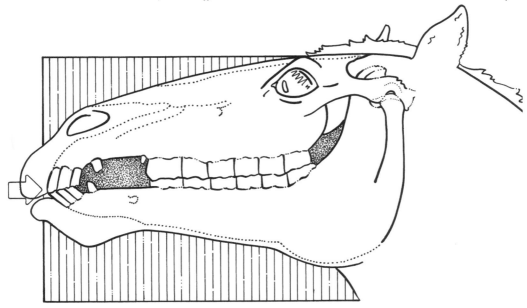

Figure 4-4. With poll flexed, the lower incisors are usually even with or slightly anterior to the upper incisors.

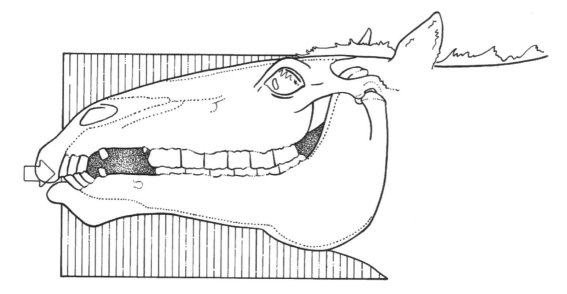

Figure 4-5. With poll extended, the upper incisors are normally further anterior than the lower incisors

Incisor Table Angle

The incisor table angle refers to the slope of the occlusal surface of the incisor arcades (viewed from the side) relative to the bars of the mouth (the dorsal surface of the mandible, between the corner incisor and the first cheek tooth). It does not refer to the angle of the teeth themselves, just to their collective occlusal surface (table). It is evaluated relative to the bars of the mouth, not to the vertical plane of the incisors (Fig. 4-6).

When viewed from the side of the horse's mouth, the incisor table normally slopes upward slightly from labial to lingual surface (i.e., from front to back) (Figs. 4-7 and 4-8). The normal incisor table angle is 10 to 15 degrees relative to the bars. Overjet or underjet can increase or decrease, respectively, the incisor table angle. I usually evaluate this angle by eye, although I have an adjustable protractor that I can use to more accurately gauge the angle. I record any deviation from normal on the dental chart before performing any work on the incisors.

Incidentally, although the incisors slope rostrally with advancing age in geriatric horses, the incisor table angle should still be 10 to 15 degrees relative to the bars in these horses. The only instances in which I have seen the incisor table angle change in geriatric horses were those in which the incisors were loose, in which case the incisor table angle was approximately 0 degrees (i.e., parallel with the bars).

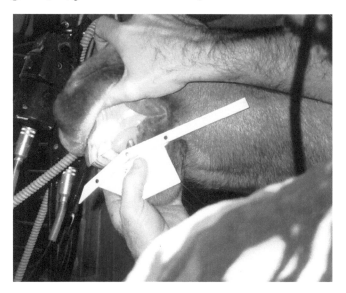

Figure 4-6. Evaluating the incisor table angle aided by a protractor set at 15 degrees.

Molar Occlusion

Evaluation of molar occlusion involves estimating the width of the molar tables, expressed as a percentage, in active occlusion during mastication. (*Molar* in this section refers to both the premolars and molars as a masticatory unit.) When dentition and mastication are normal, molar occlusion should be 90% to 100%, meaning that almost the entire width of the molar occlusal surface is involved in grinding foodstuffs during the "power stroke" of mastication.

The power stroke involves the lower molars sliding across the upper molars, in a buccal-to-palatal (lateral-to-medial) direction, once the upper and lower jaws are brought together. The molar table normally has an angle of 12 to 15 degrees from horizontal, with the slope running down toward the buccal surface, so the lower molars normally move both medially and dorsally (i.e., toward the palate) as they slide across the uppers (Fig. 4-9). (Horses chew predominantly on one side of the mouth at a time, periodically alternating from left to right sides.)

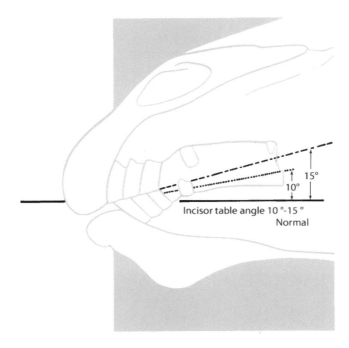

Figure 4-7. Normal incisor table angle at 10 to 15 degrees.

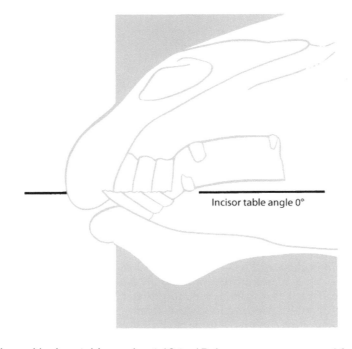

Figure 4-8. Normal incisor table angle at 10 to 15 degrees as measured from the bars.

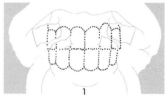

Mouth closed, not chewing. (This horse has approximately 75% molar occlusion.)

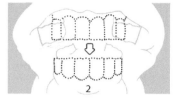

Dropping lower jaw to begin chewing. Tongue and/or cheek places grass or hay on molar table.

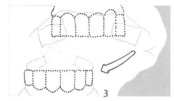

Lower jaw moves to the side in which chewing will occur.

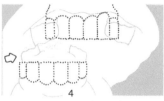

Jaw moves up and in to begin power stroke.

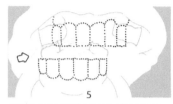

Mid power stroke (up and in along normal 15° molar table angle).

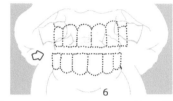

Lower arcades continue up and in until incisors meet. (The cycle continues, perhaps switching sides periodically, unless painful malocclusions encourage one-sided chewing.)

Figure 4-9. Mastication sequence.

Several factors can interfere with this process, limiting the full extent of molar occlusion and resulting in abnormal wear of the molar tables (see Chapter 5). Uncorrected, low molar occlusion eventually leads to abnormal tooth wear and problems with mastication. The method I use for evaluating molar occlusion consists of two parts: (1) lateral excursion test, and (2) visual examination of molar contact.

Lateral Excursion Test for Molar Occlusion

This test is best performed with the horse sedated so resistance by the masticatory muscles is minimal (Fig. 4-10). It is performed with the horse's jaws closed (incisors meeting), but with the horse's lips gently parted (using your thumbs or fingers) so that the incisors can be visualized during the test. With one hand over the bridge of the horse's nose and the other hand under the mandible, just behind the horse's chin, slide the mandible to one side until resistance is met. While doing so, observe the vertical line between the central incisors on the lower arcade (301 and 401). Note the position of this line relative to the upper incisors at the following two key points in its excursion:

1. When the incisors separate (which is the point at which the molars come into occlusion)
2. At the furthest extent of mandibular excursion (i.e., when resistance is met) (Figs. 4-11 to 4-15)

At the starting point (neutral position), the line between 301 and 401 should match the line between 101 and 201 (unless the mandible or the maxilla is crooked, in which case begin by noting the position of the line between the lower centrals relative to the upper centrals).* When molar occlusion is 90% to 100%, which is ideal, the incisors separate at almost the moment the mandible is slid laterally from the starting position.

This method for estimating the percentage of molar occlusion is illustrated in the following example. If the lower line has traversed two incisor widths at maximum excursion (point 2), but had traveled halfway across the central incisor when the incisors separated (point 1), molar occlusion is approximately 75%. In this example, the molars are *not* in occlusion for 25% of the maximum mandibular excursion—half an incisor width out of a maximum distance of two incisor widths (one quarter, or 25%). So, molar occlusion is 75%.

Some dental practitioners advocate estimating these distances in fractions of an inch or in millimeters, rather than as incisor widths. Whichever method you use, it is important to express the result of the lateral excursion test as a *percentage*—point 1 relative to point 2—rather than as a fixed distance. Doing so eliminates the variable of incisor size between horses of differing age, breed, and height. (NOTE: The maximum distance of lateral excursion, measured in incisor widths, may be greater in geriatric horses than in younger horses because the teeth of older horses are narrower.)

Be sure to slide the mandible in both directions (to the left and to the right) and estimate molar occlusion for each side of the mouth; it is not always identical. Record the percentage of molar occlusion for each side of the mouth on the dental chart before performing any dental work.

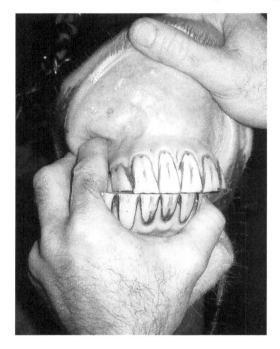

Figure 4-10. Hand position for the lateral excursion test to determine molar occlusion. (Courtesy Joe Allen, Edinboro, PA.)

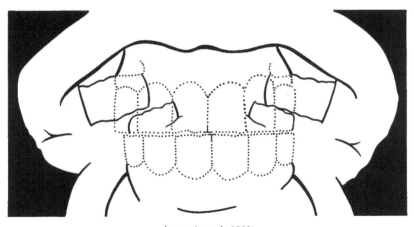

Approximately 100%
lateral excursion test for molar occlusion

Figure 4-11. Lateral excursion test picturing 100% molar occclusion

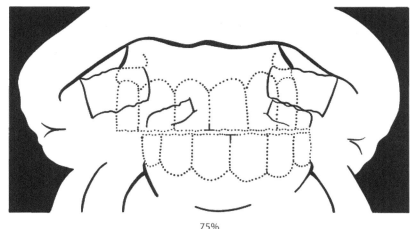

75%
Lateral excursion test for molar occlusion

Figure 4-12. Lateral excursion test picturing 75% molar occlusion.

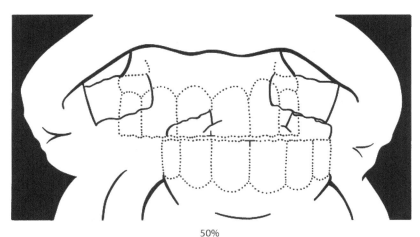

50%
Lateral excursion test for molar occlusion

Figure 4-13. Lateral excursion test picturing 50% molar occlusion.

It is important to understand that this test only estimates the *width* of the molar occlusal surface that is in contact with the opposing arcade during mastication. It does not evaluate the *length* (rostral-caudal distance) of the molar table that is in occlusion. The horse may have only one pair of teeth (one upper and one lower) in occlusion on a particular side, but if they are wearing evenly, molar occlusion, as assessed by the lateral excursion test, may be close to 100%. Clearly, this single measurement can be misleading without visual examination of molar contact.

Visual Examination of Molar Contact

This simple assessment is performed with the patient's jaws closed, using a cheek retractor and a good light source (Figs. 4-16 to 4-19). It involves drawing the cheek laterally (away from the cheek teeth) with the retractor and visually examining the buccal aspect of the molar arcades for gaps between upper and lower teeth—areas along the length of the molar table where any of the teeth are not in occlusion.

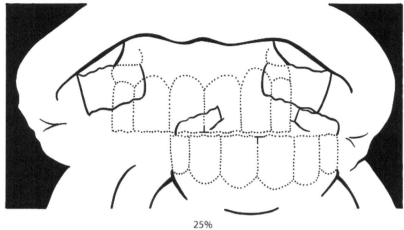

25%
Lateral excursion test for molar occlusion

Figure 4-14. Lateral excursion test picturing 25% molar occlusion.

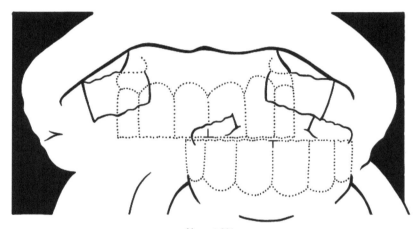

Almost 0%
Lateral excursion test for molar occlusion

Figure 4-15. Lateral excursion test picturing almost 0% molar occlusion.

The most commonly encountered, but least recognized, cause of defective occlusion is overly long incisors, which prevent the upper and lower cheek teeth from meeting or effectively grinding during mastication (see Chapter 5). The most commonly *recognized* cause of defective occlusion is a missing or malaligned tooth. During the next part of the examination, in which a full-mouth speculum is used, the molar tables are visually examined for irregularities that might reduce effective occlusal surface area.

ORAL EXAMINATION USING A SPECULUM

Fitting the Full-Mouth Speculum

If the patient has not already been sedated, I generally administer a sedative before applying the full-mouth speculum. If the patient's head has been supported in a dental frame for the preceding evaluations, the head is removed from the dental frame before the speculum is fitted.

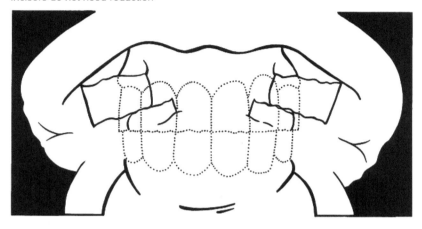

A/P view
Non-supplemented horse
Molar contact
Incisors do not need reduction

Figure 4-16. Anteroposterior (AP) view; nonsupplemented (grazing for all nutrition, receiving no grain or hay supplementation to the diet) horse showing molar contact and incisors that do not need reduction.

I use the following technique to fit the speculum: With the palm of one hand supporting the incisor plates of the speculum against the horse's incisors, insert the thumb or fingers of the same hand into the interdental space, just caudal to the incisors, and gently apply upward pressure to the maxilla (Color Plate 33). (Support the speculum with the other hand by holding up the poll strap using the back of the hand.) Unless the horse is unable to open its mouth because of pain or some other extraordinary circumstance, this gentle action is sufficient to encourage the horse to part its jaws. The incisor plates can then be slipped between the upper and lower incisors, and the poll strap secured.

Before opening the jaws of the speculum, make sure the incisor plates are properly positioned between the horse's upper and lower incisors and the poll strap is secured snugly. Also make sure the nose band on the horse's head collar or halter is loose enough to allow the horse's mouth to be opened fully. Alternatively, before fitting the speculum, undo the poll strap of the halter, slip the nose band off the horse's nose, and refasten the poll strap around the horse's neck. When opening the horse's mouth with the speculum, *do so gradually,* allowing the horse's masseter muscles time to relax and thus better accommodate the speculum. Also ensure that the speculum is open the same amount on both sides of the mouth.

An assistant, a dental stand or crutch, a dental frame, a dental halter, or a rope attached to the suspension bar of the speculum can support the head of the sedated patient. With the speculum open, briefly look into the patient's mouth. If any feed obscures visibility, rinse out the mouth with water using a large dosing syringe (Fig. 4-20). Make sure the patient's chin is lower than the base of the tongue before rinsing out the mouth, so the water flows out the mouth rather than toward the pharynx. I catch the rinse in a plastic bucket to avoid soaking the work area at my feet or wetting any electrical connections.

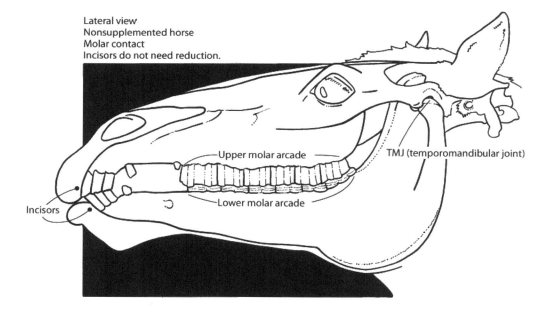

Figure 4-17. Lateral view; nonsupplemented horse showing molar contact and incisors that do not need reduction.

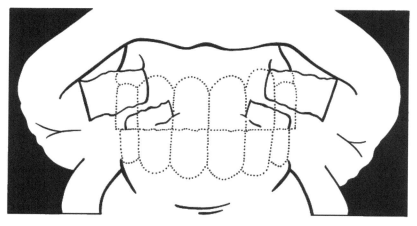

Figure 4-18. AP view; supplemented horse showing less molar contact and incisors that need reduction.

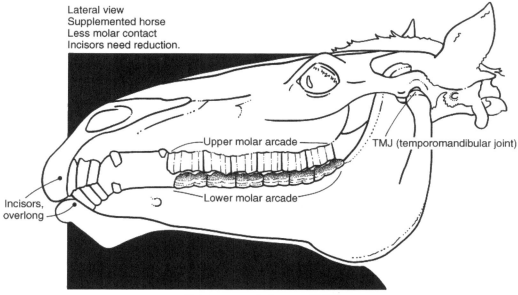

Lateral view
Supplemented horse
Less molar contact
Incisors need reduction.

Upper molar arcade

TMJ (temporomandibular joint)

Lower molar arcade

Incisors, overlong

All pressure on incisors and TMJs

Figure 4-19. Lateral view; supplemented horse showing less molar contact and incisors that need reduction.

Examination of the Canine Teeth

The number and condition of the canine teeth should be noted on the dental chart. There is sexual dimorphism associated with the canine teeth in horses. Mares often have unerupted canine teeth. The canine teeth most likely to be erupted in mares are the lowers, and their crowns typically are small (8 to 10mm long). It is common for older geldings and stallions to have long, sharp canine teeth; the uppers may be short but they can have very sharp edges.

Examine the ventral aspect of the tongue in horses with long lower canine teeth. It is common to find ulcerated areas or evidence of scarring from previous damage caused by these teeth. In older horses, the lower canine teeth are often encased in masses of tartar that may be up to 2cm thick. The surrounding gum usually is inflamed and bleeds a little when the tartar is removed (Fig. 4-21, Color Plate 34).

Examination of the Wolf Teeth

Wolf teeth are the usually small first premolars (the 5s), located in the space between the canine and the cheek teeth, just rostral to the first cheek teeth (the 6s). Wolf teeth usually erupt in horses between 6 and 12 months of age. However, not all horses have fully formed wolf teeth; and in those that do have wolf teeth, not all of these teeth fully erupt. Erupted wolf teeth are most often found in the upper arcades (105 and 205); occasionally they are also found in the lower arcades (305 and 405). There is no sexual dimorphism associated with the wolf teeth; they are found in males and females with equal frequency (Color Plate 35).

Unerupted ("blind") wolf teeth can be more of a problem than erupted wolf teeth because they may irritate the overlying gum and be irritated by the bit. They are detected as a firm nodule under the gum, located a little further rostral than is usual for erupted wolf teeth (i.e., 1 to 2cm rostral to the 6s). They are most common in the upper arcades (Color Plate 36).

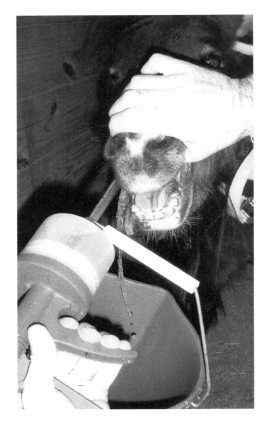

Figure 4-20. The mouth can be rinsed with the speculum in place.

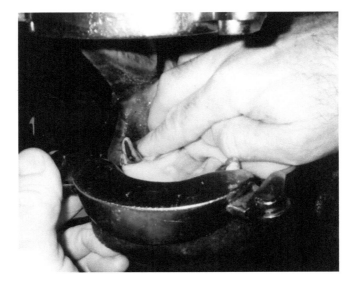

Figure 4-21. Long, sharp canines

Blind wolf teeth are easily missed if the gums are not palpated. Thus it is important to visually inspect the mouth *and palpate the gum* just rostral to the 6s in all four quadrants (upper and lower, left and right). Note the presence and location of any wolf teeth on the dental chart.

Bone spurs may also be found on the bars (the lower interdental spaces) as a result of damage to the periodontal covering of the bone there.

Examination of the Soft Tissues

Examine the tongue, cheeks, lips, gums, and palate, noting any abnormalities on the dental chart. Ulcerations or lacerations on the buccal mucosa and tongue, scars, cysts, melanomas, and polyps are among the more common findings. Occasionally, pinpoint areas of ulceration are found in the oral mucosa, in association with bot fly larvae.

Buccal Ulceration

Buccal lacerations and ulcerations are commonly found adjacent to sharp enamel points on the buccal margins of the upper cheek teeth. These ulcerated areas usually are obvious when examining the cheek adjacent to the upper 6s to 9s with a good light source (Color Plate 37). To examine the buccal mucosa adjacent to the upper 10s and 11s, it is often necessary to retract the cheek laterally using a cheek retractor or a long, blunt screwdriver. It is also important to palpate the buccal mucosa adjacent to these caudal teeth, because good visualization can be difficult, particularly in horses with thick masseter muscles (e.g., quarter horses, stallions of any breed).

I note the location and severity of buccal ulcerations on the dental chart and estimate the size of the ulcerated area in square centimeters. In addition, I record the apparent depth of the ulcerated areas (based on visual appearance) as abrasions only, deep, or very deep.

Examination of the Cheek Teeth Arcades

Bit Seats

Forming a bit seat refers to the practice of rounding the rostral occlusal margin of the first cheek teeth (Color Plate 38) (see Chapter 5). Because many equine dental practitioners routinely form bit seats on most or all of their patients, finding a well-formed bit seat in an adult horse you are examining for the first time is an indication that the horse has received dental care in the past 12 months. (In horses 2 to 3 years of age, the bit seat is "lost" when the deciduous first cheek teeth are shed, so absence of a bit seat cannot be taken to indicate absence of thorough dental care in this age group.)

Molar Table Angles

The molar table angle refers to the angle of the occlusal surface of the premolars and molars relative to the horizontal plane. On the lower arcades, the molar table normally slopes downward 12 to 15 degrees from lingual to buccal margin. The upper arcades have a corresponding angle from palatal to buccal margin. That is, the lower molars are slightly longer at their inner edge, and the upper molars are slightly longer at their outer edge (Fig. 4-22).

This angulation presumably results from the disparity in width of the upper and lower jaws, the upper jaw being a little wider than the lower jaw. Certain conditions cause the molar table angles to be substantially different from normal, such as 0 degrees (level) in horses with low molar occlusion, or more than 40 degrees in horses with shear mouth (see Chapter 5).

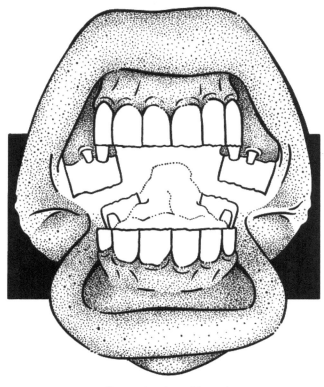

Sharp points, buccal/lingual
12-15° molar table angle

Figure 4-22. Twelve-to fifteen-degree molar table angle, AP view.

I estimate the molar table angle and record it on the dental chart before performing any work on the molars. Although the molar table angle can be estimated by eye, an adjustable protractor can be used to more accurately gauge the molar table angle. I hold the protractor between my eye and the horse's mouth, such that it overlies the molar arcade I am evaluating (Fig. 4-23). Because it is difficult to measure the molar table angle of the upper arcades in this manner, I simply measure the angle of each lower arcade (which mirrors that of the corresponding upper arcade).

The molar table angle is not uniform along the length of the molar arcade; it may increase a couple of degrees from the first cheek tooth to the last, especially in horses with narrow heads. In human dentistry, this normal and gradual change in angle is called the *curvature of Wilson*. Its significance in equine dentistry is not known. I currently estimate the molar table angle at two places along the molar arcade: at the 7s and at the 10s, noting the angle at each level on the dental chart.

Curve of Spee

This normal anatomic feature refers to the slight dorsoventral curvature of the maxilla and mandible, and thus the tables of the molar arcades, along their length. A more pronounced curve of Spee is found in breeds with "dished" faces, such as Arabians and miniature horses (Fig. 4-24). The slight ventral curvature (bulge) of the maxilla, and thus of the upper molar arcade, is reflected in a corresponding slight ventral curvature (dip) in the lower molar arcade, at about midarcade (8s and 9s). This normal anatomic feature should not be misinterpreted as wave mouth nor as dominant or overpowering upper 8s, 9s, or 10s (see Chapter 5).

In many horses, the gentle curve of the lower molar arcade concludes with the occlusal surfaces of the lower 10s and 11s sloping up slightly from front to back. The curvature of the mandible at this point also contributes to the slope of these last two teeth. This normal anatomic feature must not be misinterpreted as ramps on the lower molars (see Chapter 5). Some horses have no such curvature (Figs. 4-25 and 4-26).

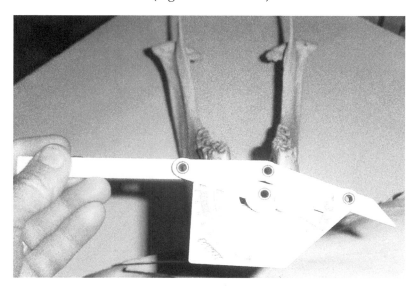

Figure 4-23. Protractor sighting molar table angles.

Problems Involving Individual Cheek Teeth

After evaluating the molar arcade as a whole, each of the teeth and the adjacent tissues should be examined. I work from rostral to caudal, beginning with the 6s and ending with the 11s in each arcade. However you decide to examine these structures, develop a system and follow it every time to ensure that your examination is thorough. Record the location and description of any abnormalities found. The following are the more common cheek teeth abnormalities I find in my equine dentistry practice:

- Upper 6 hooks—elongation of the rostral margin of the upper 6s
- Lower 6 ramps—elongation of the rostral margin of the lower 6s
- Sharp enamel points (see later discussion)
- Retained deciduous premolars—caps that are not shed when the underlying permanent tooth erupts or attempts to erupt
- Wave mouth—excessive undulation of the molar tables (e.g., a hump in the center of the lower arcade and a corresponding "hollowed out" section in the upper arcade)
- Excessive transverse ridges—taller-than-normal ridges of premolars or molars that run across the occlusal surface
- Cupped-out upper 9s—concavity of the occlusal surface of the expiring upper 9s
- Fractured upper 9s (see later discussion)
- Steps—sudden change in molar table height, caused by elongation of one or two teeth
- Shear mouth—greatly increased molar table angle
- Loose or missing teeth (see later discussion)
- Periodontal pockets (see later discussion)
- Upper 11 hooks—elongation of the caudal margin of the upper 11s
- Lower 11 ramps—elongation of the caudal margin of the lower 11s

Each of these abnormalities is discussed in Chapter 5. However, a few comments pertaining to examination findings are in order here.

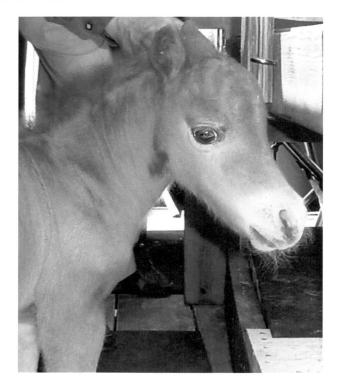

Figure 4-24. Miniature horses and Arabians often have accentuated curve of Spee.

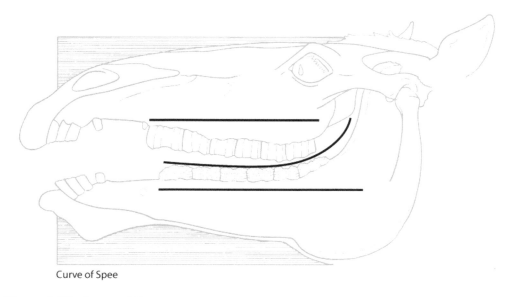

Curve of Spee

Figure 4-25. Curve of Spee.

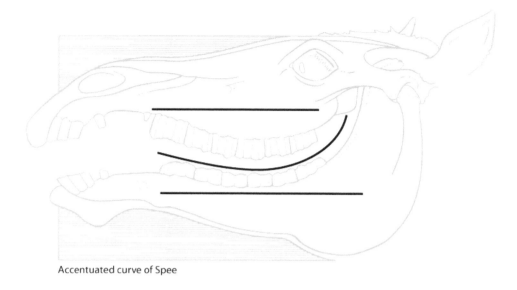

Accentuated curve of Spee

Figure 4-26. Accentuated curve of Spee.

Sharp Enamel Points

Sharp enamel points are commonly found at the margin of the occlusal surface on the buccal side of the upper cheek teeth and the lingual side of the lower cheek teeth (Fig. 4-27). Using a full-mouth speculum, these enamel points can be identified by sight, but their presence and impact are better appreciated by feeling along the margins of the molar tables with the fingers.[*]

A common misconception is that these sharp enamel points protrude beyond the level of the occlusal plane. Careful visual inspection of the molar tables shows that in most cases the enamel points do not protrude; it only *feels* as if they do. The prominence of these enamel points is a function of two anatomic features: (1) the acute angle between the occlusal surface and the vertical face of the tooth (owing to the natural angle of the molar tables), and (2) the vertical folds on the buccal (upper arcade) and lingual (lower arcade) surfaces of the teeth (Color Plate 39).

These vertical folds, or *cingula*, are most prominent on the buccal surface of the upper cheek teeth. The deeper they are, the more prominent (and sharp) are the enamel points. The sharpness of the enamel points, and thus their ability to lacerate the adjacent buccal mucosa, is also related to cementum wear from the outer surface of the tooth. As the periodontal cementum wears away, it leaves a sharp, brittle ridge of enamel at the outer margin of the occlusal surface.

In addition to noting the location of the sharpest points on the upper cheek teeth, I estimate the size of the most prominent points (in millimeters) and record it on the dental chart. Because the prominence of the enamel points is, in part, a function of the depth of the vertical folds, I am basically estimating the amount of enamel (and cementum) that lies beyond the intersection between the occlusal plane and the vertical plane at the base of the folds (Fig. 4-28). (In other words, I am estimating the amount of marginal enamel and cementum between the peaks and valleys of the vertical folds.)

Sagittally Fractured Upper 9s

Fractures of the cheek teeth are relatively uncommon. Most common is sagittal fracture of an upper 9 (109 or 209). As these teeth begin to reach the end of their useful life, they become cupped out and weakened (see Chapter 5). Masticatory forces may be sufficient to split them sagittally (parallel with the long axis of the molar table) (Color Plate 40).

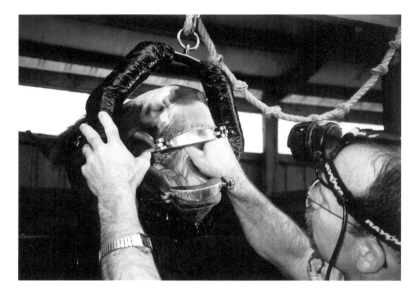

Figure 4-27. Using a full-mouth speculum and a light source, enamel points can be identified by sight. (From Allen T: Equine dentistry demand for dental care is on the rise; can you deliver? DVM News Magazine 32(9):1, 2001.)

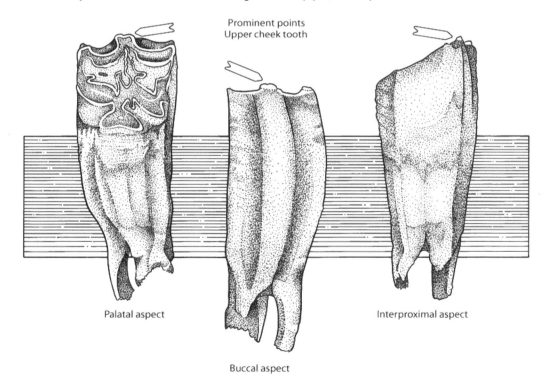

Figure 4-28. Length of sharp points on a tooth.

Typically the lateral half of the fractured tooth is found leaning out toward the buccal mucosa, and the medial half is found tilting toward the palate, often interfering with mastication. Amazingly, the patient usually shows no obvious signs of dental fracture or irritation by the fracture fragments. However, if apical infection has extended into the maxillary sinus, a malodorous unilateral nasal discharge may be noted.

Loose Teeth

Occasionally, loose cheek teeth are immediately obvious, because they fall out when the mouth is held open by the full-mouth speculum. Evidently, horses in these cases cannot or do not open their mouths wide enough or long enough for the loose teeth to fall out and be lost. However, most loose teeth are not so easily identified. Manipulation with the fingers or application of a little force with some type of probe (e.g., a long, blunt screwdriver) is necessary to identify loose cheek teeth that are held snugly in place between adjacent teeth.

Loose teeth in the upper arcades usually are easy to identify. The last couple of teeth in the lower arcade are more difficult to assess, especially if they are hidden behind a large step or wave. It is best to palpate these teeth for excessive movement. With the full-mouth speculum secured, I reach in and palpate each of the lower cheek teeth in turn, applying force across the tooth (in a buccal–palatal-lingual direction).

Some loose cheek teeth are not identified during this initial examination because they are wedged securely between adjacent teeth. It is only after dental work with power equipment that these teeth are seen to be abnormal. Following removal of the surface debris with rinsing and application of a motorized burr or float, exudate may be seen between the loose tooth and the adjacent tooth, having been vibrated to the surface by the action of the burr. Being able to visualize the teeth during the initial examination and as the work is being done is an important benefit of using a full-mouth speculum, rather than working "blind" (see Chapter 6).

(Note: With advancing age, the reserve crown of the cheek teeth becomes shorter and narrower, resulting in a smaller surface area for the periodontal ligament to anchor the tooth in the socket. Thus the cheek teeth in geriatric horses are easier to move, which should be taken into consideration when evaluating the molar arcades for pathologically loose teeth.)

Periodontal Pockets

Various malocclusive conditions may force the cheek teeth apart, allowing food particles to pack into the gap between the teeth, forming an abnormally large space between the teeth called a *diastema*. Pressure on the underlying gingiva and periodontal bone may cause inflammation and eventually necrosis of these tissues. A pocket forms between the tooth and the bone that readily becomes packed with food particles, exacerbating the process. Pockets between the gums and teeth are called periodontal pockets.

These pockets are most commonly found, and are easiest to detect, in the upper arcades, presumably because lower waves (which overpower the corresponding upper cheek teeth) are the most commonly encountered type of malocclusion. Periodontal pockets may also form in the lower arcades, so both upper and lower arcades should be thoroughly examined. It is usually necessary to hold the tongue to the opposite side to inspect the lingual aspects of the lower cheek teeth. I have a set of dental picks at various angles that I use for exploring the periodontal area if visual inspection suggests a periodontal pocket. Periodontal disease is discussed further in Chapter 7 (Color Plate 41).

Missing Teeth

Lost cheek teeth are common in older horses. Often the first indication of a missing tooth is overgrowth of the opposing tooth, resulting in a step in the opposing arcade. It is important to check the gum carefully for fragments of the tooth or its root when spaces are found in the molar arcades.

COMPLETION OF THE EXAMINATION

Once the examination is complete, ensure that all routinely evaluated indices and abnormal findings are recorded on the dental chart. Discuss the significance of any findings with the owner or agent, then make appropriate recommendations for dental correction. If the owner chooses not to have any dental work performed at that time, I administer a reversal agent (see Chapter 3) so that the patient will be sufficiently alert and coordinated to be safely moved out of the work area. If the owner or agent gives permission to proceed with the recommended dental work, I do not use the reversal agent until the work is completed.

RECOMMENDED READING

The following references are recommended for an in-depth review of dental anatomy:

Dixon PM: Dental anatomy. In Baker GJ, Easley J, editors: Equine dentistry, London, 1999, WB Saunders.
Easley J: Equine dental development and anatomy. Proceedings of the forty-second annual convention of the American Association of Equine Practitioners, Lexington, KY, 1996.
Lowder MQ, Mueller POE: Dental embryology, anatomy, development, and aging, Vet Clin North Am Equine Pract 14:227, 1999.

* *It is relatively common for the line between 301 and 401 to be a little to one side of the line between 101 and 201. When the two center lines do not match, make a note on the dental chart, indicating the exact position of the lower center line relative to 101-201 in the neutral, or resting, position. For example, write "lowers centered at one-third width of 101," or "lowers centered at one-half width of 201."*

* *Many practitioners determine the presence and relevance of sharp enamel points simply by pressing the horse's cheeks against the outer margins of the upper cheek teeth while the horse's mouth is closed. If the horse raises its head, pulls away, or shows some other type of evasive behavior, the conclusion is that the horse needs its teeth floated. If the horse does not appear to resent this maneuver, the presumption is the horse's teeth are all right.*

This approach is to be discouraged for a couple of reasons. First, because this procedure can cause the horse pain when sharp enamel points dig into the buccal mucosa, I think it is incumbent upon the practitioner to select a more humane means of evaluating the horse's teeth. Second, because sharp enamel points are only one of several possible abnormalities that commonly involve the teeth caudal to the commissures of the lips, and because it is not possible to thoroughly examine the horse's mouth without the aid of a full-mouth speculum and a good light source, this procedure is grossly inadequate for determining the need for dental care.

Virtually all horses that have not received thorough dental care in the past 3 to 12 months will have sharp enamel points, regardless of whether the horse reacts to digital pressure on the cheeks overlying these areas. A far better approach is to advise the owner or caretaker that thorough examination of the mouth is required to determine whether the horse needs dental care. If it is not convenient for the practitioner to conduct the examination at that time, an appointment can be made for a more suitable time.

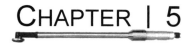

CHAPTER 5

Common Dental Abnormalities

Before discussing correction of dental abnormalities, it is important to discuss why certain findings are considered abnormal and in need of correction. Fractured teeth, grossly misshapen or malaligned teeth, and loose or missing permanent teeth are obviously abnormal. Other less dramatic findings generally are considered problematic because practitioners surmise or have observed that they adversely affect dental function or cause the animal discomfort. There is considerable debate among equine practitioners as to whether certain findings constitute an abnormality that requires correction, and if so, how much intervention is required. For this reason, an equine dental paradigm is proposed as a standard for equine dental care (Fig. 5-1).

EQUINE DENTAL PARADIGM

Dale Jeffrey and Tom Allen

A paradigm is a model or a frame of reference; a set of parameters that defines a particular concept. The equine dental paradigm uses observations and measurements equine practitioners interpret as normal for equine dentition as the ideal for which to strive when performing equine dental procedures (Figs. 5-2 to 5-10). In essence, practitioners endeavor to normalize specific dental elements in a patient judged to have abnormal dentition (with the under standing that certain severe or long-standing abnormalities may not be amenable to complete correction).

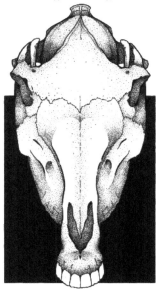

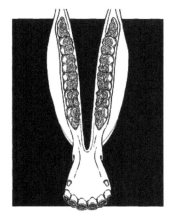

| Dorsal view, skull | Ventrodorsal intraoral view | Dorsoventral intraoral view |

Figure 5-1. **A**, Dorsal view of the skull. **B**, Ventrodorsal view. **C**, Dorsoventral intraoral view

Defining Normal

Establishing this paradigm begins with defining what is normal. Because very little research has been conducted on equine dental structure and function, developing an equine dental paradigm must begin with some basic assumptions:

1. The population from which the specifications of normal equine dentition are derived consists of healthy horses grazing grass and other living plant material—that is, the diet for which this species is evolutionarily adapted—as their sole source of nourishment.
2. The structure and orientation of the teeth in the normal equine mouth serve a specific purpose in maintaining the animal's health and well-being, even if we have not yet ascertained the specific purpose. (As the architectural adage goes, form follows function.)
3. Some of the parameters that define normal must cover a range to account for individual variation among normal animals and differences related to geographic region.

So, what is normal dentition in a healthy horse whose dietary intake is derived solely from grazing? Based on our observations, made over two decades and many thousands of equine mouths, the following can be expected in the mouth of an adult horse that has not undergone any dental procedures:

- There is at least 6 mm of rostral-caudal excursion of the mandible relative to the maxilla.[*]
- The incisor arcades meet in a horizontal line (taking into account the curved rostral contour of the upper and lower jaws) as viewed from the front.
- The incisor table angle is 10 to 15 degrees, relative to the bars of the mouth.[*]
- In males, the canine teeth are long and sharp; in the few mares with erupted canines, the canine teeth may be sharp.
- Wolf teeth may be present on both sides of the upper arcades (105-205); less commonly, one or both upper wolf teeth are unerupted ("blind"); uncommonly, wolf teeth are present in the lower arcades (305-405).
- The cheek teeth are uniform in height along the entire molar arcade (taking into account the gentle curve of Spee), usually having taller clinical crowns toward the rostral portions of the cheek teeth arcades.
- The molar table angles are 12 to 15 degrees relative to the horizontal plane.[*]
- Molar occlusion is 90% to 100% on both sides of the mouth.[*]
- Sharp enamel points are found at the perimeter of the occlusal surface on the buccal aspect of the upper cheek teeth and possibly on the lingual aspect of the lower cheek teeth.
- The rostral contour of the 6s is block-shaped (i.e., the vertical face of the tooth meets the occlusal surface at a right angle, rather than having a rounded contour).

Because these are the parameters found in the majority of healthy adult horses eating a natural diet, *this is the model we strive to emulate* when performing corrective dental work—*with some modifications* designed to maximize the animal's comfort, particularly in horses that must wear a bit. In our experience, excessively sharp canine teeth and sharp enamel points on the upper cheek teeth often cause lacerations of the tongue and buccal mucosa, respectively. At the very least, these lacerations are likely to be painful, so the offending sharp dental elements should be remodeled or removed in any horse in which they are found. It could also be argued that removal of the wolf teeth (whether erupted or "blind") and rounding of the rostral margin of the 6s (forming a "bit seat"; see pp. 119–121) are in the horse's best interest if a bit is used to control the horse. Also, rounding the rostral portions of the 6s facilitates the entrance of long stems into the area where mastication occurs.

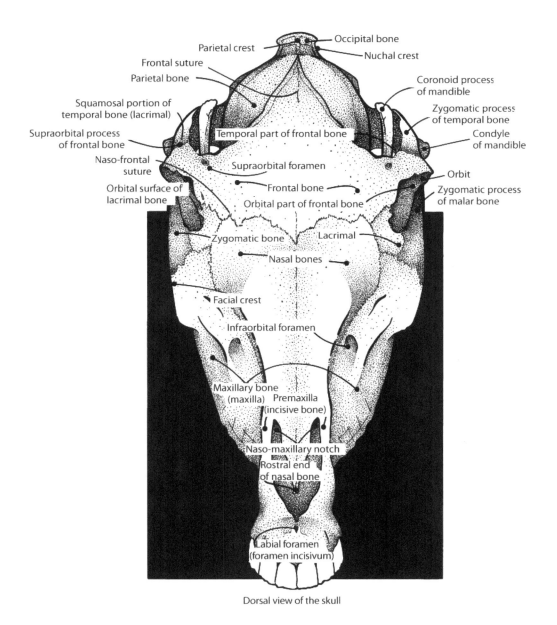

Figure 5-2. Dorsal view of the skull.

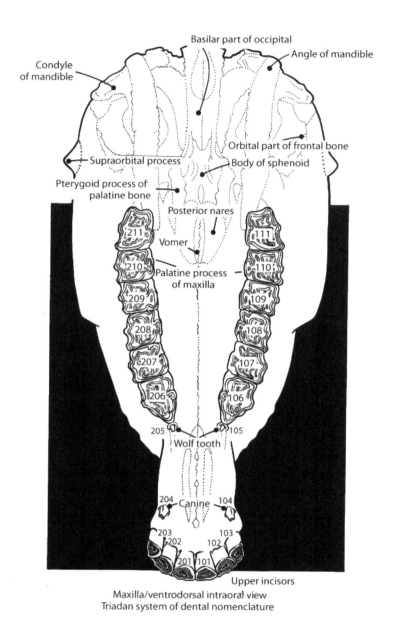

Figure 5-3. Maxilla-ventrodorsal intraoral view, —using the Triadan system of dental nomenclature.

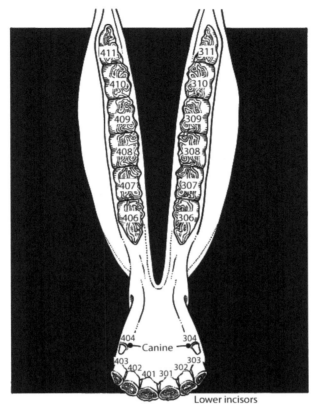

Mandible/dorsoventral intraoral view
Triadan system of dental nomenclature

Figure 5-4. Mandible-dorsoventral intraoral view, using the Triadan system of dental nomenclature.

Basis for Determining Abnormal

In this discussion of normal versus abnormal, it is important to note the distinction between *normal* and *common*. In our experience, dental overgrowths and malocclusions are *common* in domesticated horses, but that does not mean these disorders are a *normal* finding in this population. (As a loose analogy, degenerative joint disease is common in athletic horses, but it could hardly be considered normal.)

The equine dental paradigm we propose is based on the findings in healthy horses whose nutritional intake is derived solely from grazing. However, the reality is that the majority of our patients do not rely on grazing to meet all of their nutritional needs. Most are fed a ration that primarily consists of hay and some type of concentrate. We believe this "artificial" diet predisposes domesticated horses to a variety of dental abnormalities, most of which are discussed later in this chapter.

Effect of Diet

Many of the abnormalities discussed later can be understood by considering the effect of the horse's natural diet on dental function and tooth wear. Along with resilient structural components such as lignin, grasses contain variable amounts of silicates. Silica is mildly abrasive (like very fine sandpaper), so grazing results in continuous wear of the incisors as the horse snips off the stalks of grass.

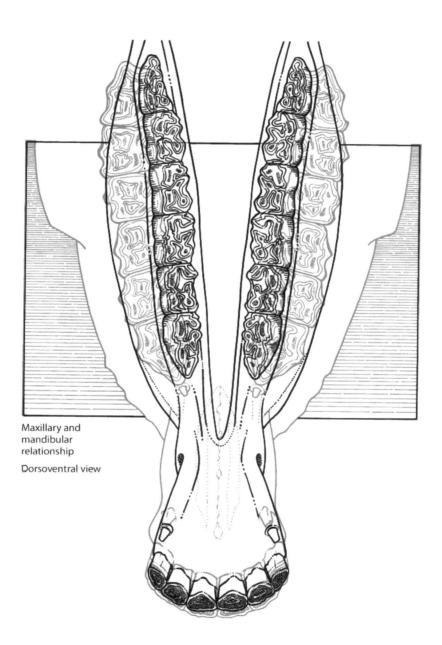

Maxillary and
mandibular
relationship

Dorsoventral view

Figure 5-5. Maxillary and mandibular relationship, dorsoventral view.

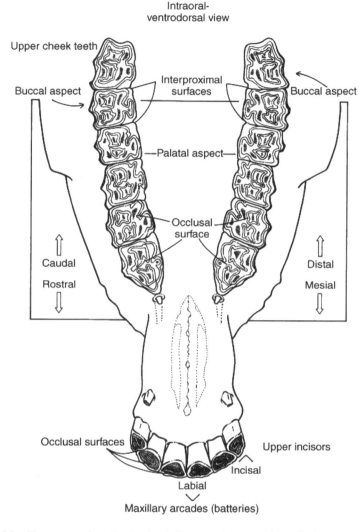

Figure 5-6. Maxillary arcades (batteries), intraoral-ventrodorsal view.

Horses fed hay as their primary roughage source do not use their incisors to prehend food to the same extent or even in the same way, so incisor wear in nongrazing horses is less than in grazing horses. As a consequence, the incisors may become overlong relative to the molar arcades, which can reduce molar occlusion, altering masticatory efficiency and contributing to abnormal wear of the molar arcades.

Dynamic Interactions

The equine dental paradigm is not limited to static observations (i.e., the structure and orientation of the teeth). It also takes into consideration the *dynamic* interactions between the maxilla and the mandible, and thus between the upper and lower dental arcades (see Fig. 5-5). Movement of the mandible in relation to the maxilla is something that can be observed and quantitated (e.g., rostral-caudal excursion of the mandible, and lateral excursion test for molar occlusion; see Chapter 4).

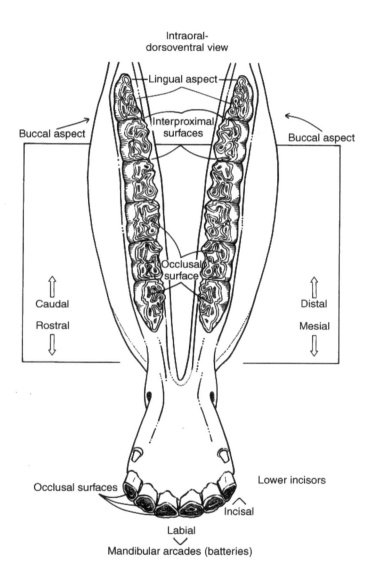

Figure 5-7. Mandibular arcades (batteries), intraoral-dorsoventral view.

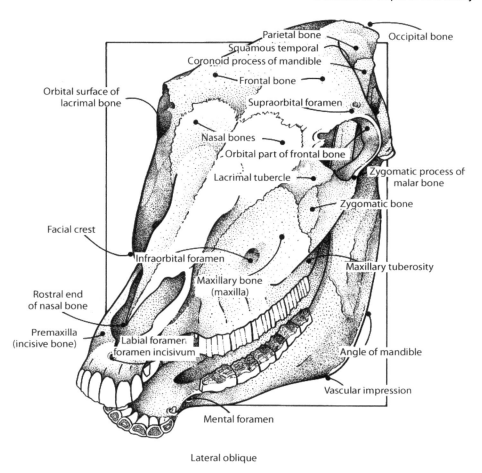

Figure 5-8. Lateral oblique view of the skull. The bony parts of the skull.

This interaction presumably is a key element of normal mastication and important in jaw movement during other activities such as locomotion. Thus, restoring a more normal relationship between the upper and lower dental arcades and normalizing balance between the left and right sides of the mouth are also important goals of dental work. In this regard, dental corrective procedures could be described as *dental equilibration.*

Goals of Dental Equilibration

The primary function of the horse's dentition is acquisition and mastication of food (Figs. 5-11 and 5-12). However, malnutrition is not the only possible outcome of dental abnormalities. As discussed in Chapter 1, dental disorders also have the potential to affect a horse's comfort, health, and athletic performance. Hence the ultimate goals of equine dental equilibration are as follows:

- Maximize the patient's comfort during mastication and athletic performance by alleviating any painful dental conditions and restoring normal rostral-caudal movement of the mandible
- Maximize masticatory efficiency by facilitating the entry and assimilation of food particles into the molar arcades
- Minimize the effects of dental disease on health and productivity by early identification and correction of dental abnormalities that impede mastication, allow oral pathogens to invade vital tissues, or accelerate dental attrition
- Optimize the biomechanics of mastication to maximize the useful life of the teeth

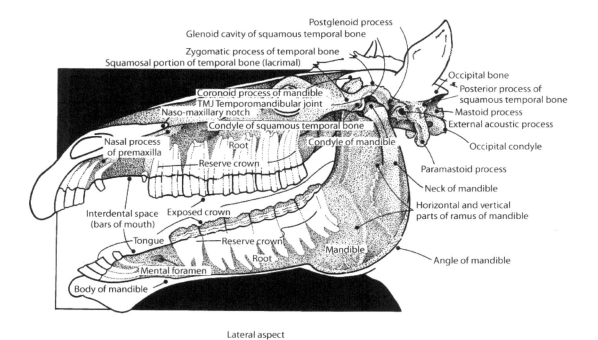

Lateral aspect

Figure 5-9. Lateral aspect of the skull. The bony parts of the skull.

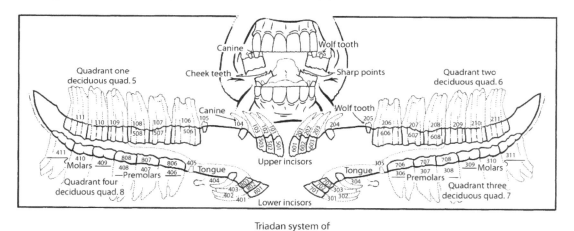

Triadan system of
dental nomenclature

Figure 5-10. Lateral view of the Triadan system of nomenclature.

The specific plan for dental equilibration should be tailored to the individual patient, factoring in the animal's age, breed, diet, environment, function, and specific dental abnormalities or propensities. Correction of the dental abnormalities discussed later in this chapter is the subject of Chapter 6.

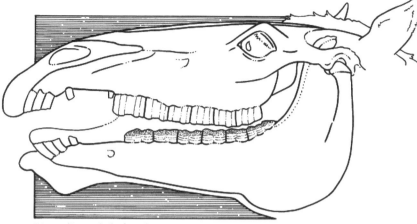

"Normal" mouth (before dentistry)

Figure 5-11. "Normal" mouth before dentistry.

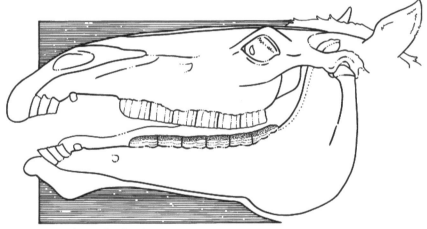

"Normal" mouth (after dentistry)

Figure 5-12. "Normal" mouth after dentistry.

INCISORS

Tom Allen

Common abnormalities involving the incisors include the following:
- Missing incisors
- Wedge or slant mouth
- Loose or damaged deciduous incisors (caps)
- Damaged permanent incisors

Less common abnormalities include supernumerary (extra) incisors, displaced inci - sors, underjet or overjet, and underbite ("hog" or "sow" mouth) or overbite ("parrot mouth") (Figs. 5-13 to 5-30).

Abnormalities of Bite and Incisor Table Angle

Overjet is an abnormality in which the labial surface of the upper incisors is further rostral than that of the lower incisors. This abnormality is not as severe as an overbite, in which the entire table of the upper incisors overlaps the lower incisors. Overjet is often associated with a greater than normal incisor table angle (see Chapter 4).

Underjet is the opposite defect: the labial surface of the lower incisors is further rostral than that of the upper incisors, but not to the extent of forming an underbite. Underjet often causes a zero or negative incisor angle (i.e., the incisor table is horizontal or slopes downward from front to back).

Although these abnormalities seem not to affect grazing ability or prehension of other foods, they can have a negative impact on molar occlusion and wear if the overlong incisors limit rostral-caudal movement or lateral excursion of the mandible. In some cases, the incisor malocclusion is accompanied by a similar disparity in the cheek teeth arcades. For example, upper 6 hooks and lower 11 ramps may be found in horses with overjets or overbites. Bite abnormalities and any associated cheek teeth malocclusions can negatively affect the horse's athletic performance by limiting rostral-caudal movement of the mandible.

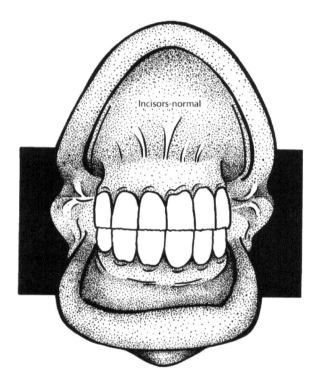

Figure 5-13. Anteroposterior (AP) view of normal incisors.

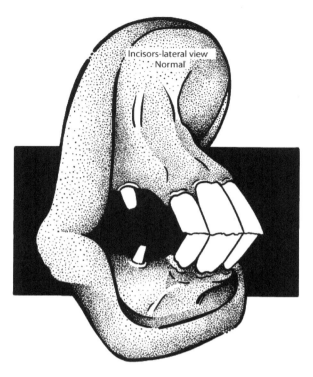

Figure 5-14. Lateral view of normal incisors.

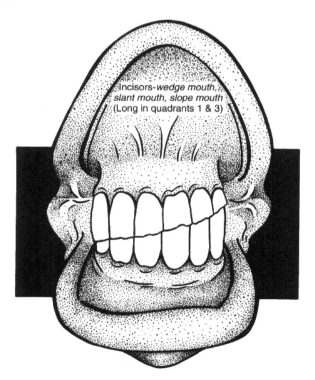

Figure 5-15. AP view. Incisors—wedge mouth, slant mouth, slope mouth, diagonal mouth. Long in quadrants 1 and 3.

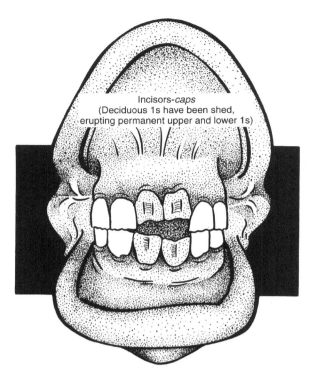

Figure 5-16. AP view. Incisors—caps. Deciduous 1s have been shed, erupting permanent upper and lower 1s.

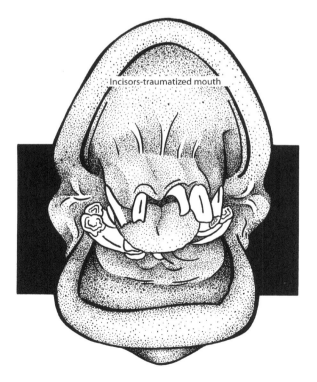

Figure 5-17. AP view. Incisors—traumatized mouth.

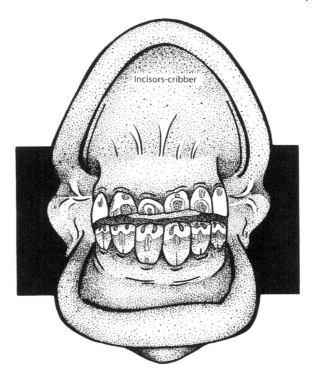

Figure 5-18. AP view. Incisors—cribber.

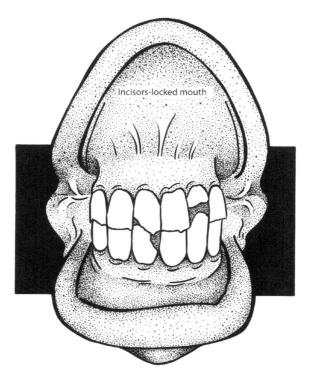

Figure 5-19. AP view. Incisors—locked mouth.

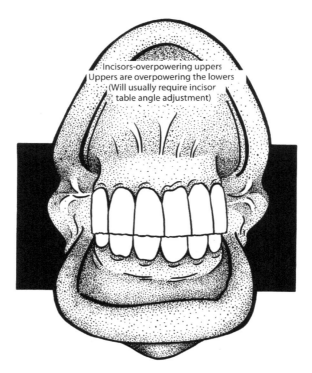

Figure 5-20. AP view. Incisors—overpowering uppers. Uppers are overpowering the lowers. This usually requires incisor table angle adjustment

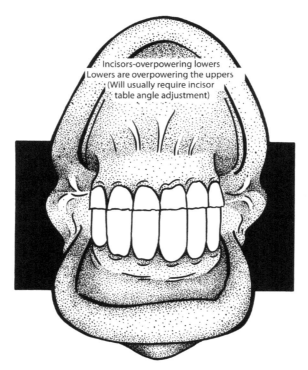

Figure 5-21. Incisors—overpowering lowers. Lowers are overpowering the uppers. This usually requires incisor table angle adjustment.

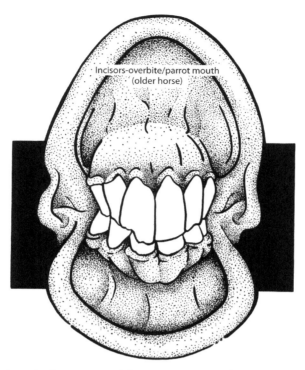

Figure 5-22. AP view. Incisors—overbite or parrot mouth on an older horse. (Upper 6 hooks, lower 11 ramps often accompany overbite.)

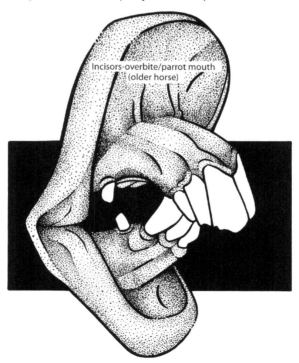

Figure 5-23. Lateral view. Incisors—overbite or parrot mouth on an older horse. (Upper 6 hooks, lower 11 ramps often accompany overbite.)

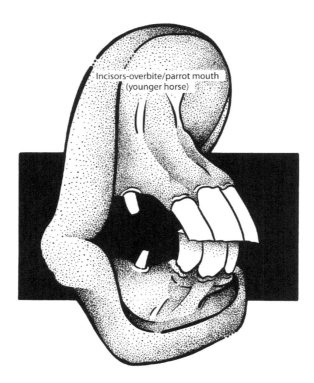

Figure 5-24. Lateral view. Incisors— overbite or parrot mouth on a younger horse. (Upper 6 hooks, lower 11 ramps often accompany overbite.)

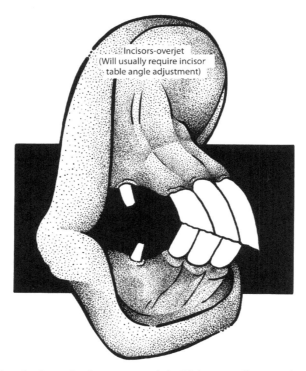

Figure 5-25. Lateral view. Incisors—overjet. This usually requires incisor table angle adjustment.

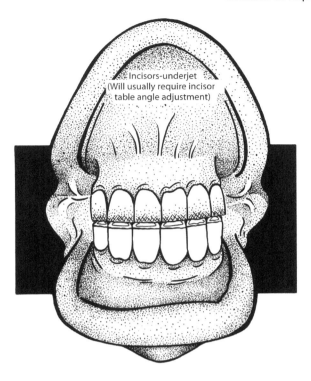

Figure 5-26. AP view. Incisors—underjet. This usually required incisor table angle adjustment.

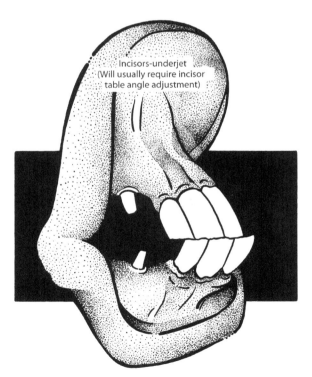

Figure 5-27. Lateral view. Incisors—underjet. This usually requires incisor table angle adjustment.

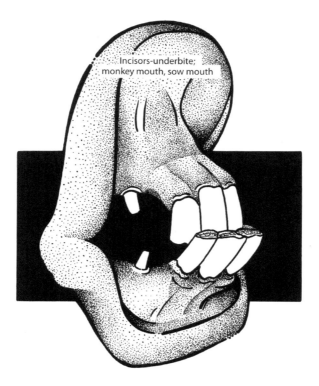

Figure 5-28. Lateral view. Incisors—underbite, monkey mouth, sow mouth.

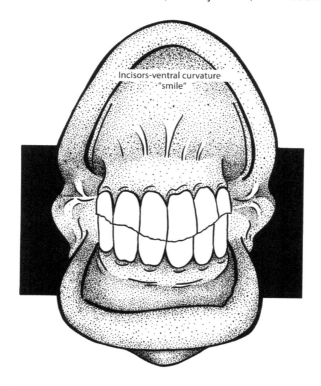

Figure 5-29. AP view. Incisors—ventral curvature, smile.

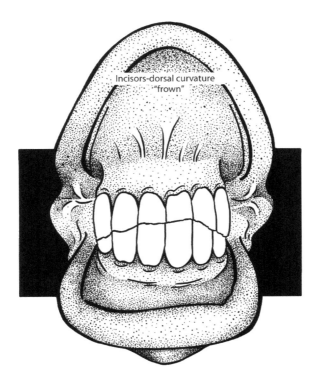

Incisors-dorsal curvature "frown"

Figure 5-30. AP view. Incisors—dorsal curvature, frown.

Incisor Line Deviations

When evaluating the incisor line for wedge or slant mouth, it is a good idea to raise the horse's chin (and/or bend your knees), until the horse's eyes line up with the incisor line. Provided the horse's head is not tilted, the eyes should be level with each other, which can be used as a horizontal marker for comparison with the incisor line.

Wedge or *slant mouth* refers to the condition in which the incisor line is straight but slopes from one side of the mouth to the other, instead of being horizontal (see Chapter 4). It usually indicates a long-standing problem on one side of the horse's mouth. Any chronic, painful condition involving the cheek teeth on one side of the mouth and ultimately leading to shear mouth (see p. 102) can result in wedge mouth, with the incisor line dropping to the same side as the shear mouth. Such conditions include loose or fractured teeth, retained caps, waves, steps, and large ramps or hooks.

Problems primarily or exclusively involving the incisors can also cause wedge mouth. Probably the most common incisor abnormality is uneven loss of deciduous incisors and/or uneven eruption of permanent incisors between the left and right sides of the mouth. It is common to find no corresponding abnormality in the cheek teeth arcades in these cases, which suggests that the wedge mouth began with an incisor abnormality.

Ventral and dorsal curvatures of the incisor line ("smiles" and "frowns") are significant because they can interfere with mastication. The upper and lower incisor arcades must be able to slide across one another during mastication, which involves a rotary action of the mandible relative to the maxilla, not just a hingelike, open-and-close motion. Overly long corner incisors (lowers with a "smile" or uppers with a "frown") can impede the movement of the lower incisors across the uppers, and thus limit molar excursion during mastication.

Any deviation from horizontal should be noted and drawn on the dental chart. With wedge mouth, the orientation of the abnormality should also be noted. For example, wedge mouth in which the incisor line is higher on the horse's left side than on the right (i.e., the line slopes down from the observer's right to left when looking at the incisors from the front) is written as *wedge mouth, long in quadrants 1 and 3.* This notation indicates that the incisors are longer on the horse's upper right (quadrant 1) and lower left (quadrant 3) (Fig. 5-31).

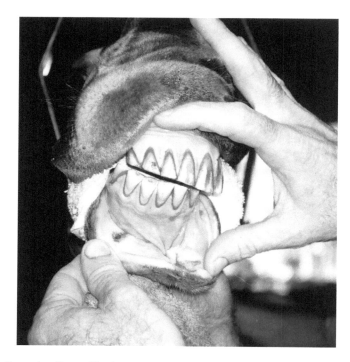

Figure 5-31. Examination of incisors commonly reveals such problems as wedge, slant, or diagonal mouth.

Incisor Length

Incisor length should be considered in relation to molar height. As discussed earlier, overlong incisors reduce the width of molar occlusion, which reduces masticatory efficiency and causes abnormal wear of the cheek teeth. For example, if the lateral excursion test indicates that molar occlusion is only 50%, only half of the molar occlusal surface is being used during mastication (see Chapter 4). One half of the occlusal surface experiences excessive wear, whereas the other half is permitted to overgrow (through the normal process of continual dental eruption). Typically, low molar occlusion results in flattening of the molar table from the normal 12- to 15-degree angle.

CANINE TEETH

The presumed role of the canine teeth in horses is self-defense, because these teeth can be quite sharp. Domesticated horses generally do not need long, sharp canine teeth for defense against predators or competitors, and they should not be allowed to cause injury to other horses, whether during fighting or play. Because sharp canine teeth can lacerate the horse's tongue or lips, blunting of the canines should be performed as a part of routine dental treatment. (Doing so also eliminates one of the potential hazards to the dental practitioner when working in a horse's mouth.)

CHEEK TEETH
Tom Allen and Dale Jeffrey

Molar Occlusion

Ideally, molar occlusion is close to 100%, meaning that virtually the entire width of the molar occlusal surface is being used during mastication. When molar occlusion is close to 100%, masticatory efficiency is maximal and the molar tables wear evenly. Several factors can reduce molar occlusion or alter molar wear, to the detriment of masticatory efficiency and molar longevity (see Figs. 4-12 to 4-16).

Incisor Length or Occlusion

The following factors can alter molar occlusion and wear by affecting incisor length or occlusion:
- Restricted grazing
- Feeding above ground level
- Stable vices (e.g., stall raking, crib biting)
- Trauma to the incisors
- Congenital defects involving the premaxilla or rostral mandible (e.g., wry mouth, parrot mouth, sow or monkey mouth)
- Other incisor malocclusions (e.g., retained deciduous teeth, locking or blocking teeth)
- Inappropriate dental care (e.g., practitioner-altered incisor table angle or crown height)

Molar Wear Patterns

The following factors can alter molar occlusion and wear:
- Trauma to one side of the head involving soft tissue, bone, muscle, and/or the TMJ
- Trauma to individual teeth (e.g., fracture and splitting of cupped-out upper 9s, biting down on a stone or other hard object while eating)
- Laceration of the buccal mucosa and/or tongue on one side of the mouth
- Supernumerary teeth
- Impacted teeth (cheek teeth wedged together so tightly that normal eruption of certain teeth is impeded; see p. 99)
- Periodontitis (see Chapter 7)

Pain on one side of the mouth or head causes the horse to chew predominantly or exclusively on the other side of the mouth. This uneven chewing pattern creates a flat table on the side being used and a more steep or exaggerated table angle (shear mouth; see p. 102) on the side being protected. It is common for horses chewing with this pattern to also limit lateral excursion during mastication. As a result, large rims or ledges may form on the buccal portions of the occlusal surfaces of the upper cheek teeth.

In addition to these "naturally occurring" factors, several man-made factors can reduce molar occlusion and/or alter the useful life of the cheek teeth:
- Artificial diet—highly digestible foods that do not require full lateral excursion of the mandible
- Dental work performed in an improper or inadequate manner (appropriate dental procedures should not prematurely age any of the teeth)
- Failure to tailor the dental treatment plan to the individual patient's needs
- Use of spool-type gags, which can lead to fracture of one or more cheek teeth
- Biting down on ill-placed floats
- Excessive tooth removal during bit seat formation or "performance" floats
- Over-floating
- Inappropriate bitting, resulting in bit wear on the rostral surfaces of the 6s

UPPER 6 HOOKS

Tom Allen

Elongation of the rostral border of the upper 6s (106, 206) is commonly called an *upper 6 hook* (Fig. 5-32). These hooks develop when the rostral border of the upper 6 is located further forward than that of the corresponding lower 6. Presumably, either the upper molar arcade is longer than the lower, or the upper and lower arcades are the same length but the lower is positioned further caudally.

The rostral portion of the upper 6 that is not being worn by the opposing lower 6 elongates as the tooth continues to erupt, and protrudes ventrally toward the bar of the mouth. In severe cases, the upper 6 hook may reach the mandible, interfering with rostral movement of the mandible during mastication and poll flexion, and causing severe pain by impinging on the soft tissue and underlying bone in the interdental space.

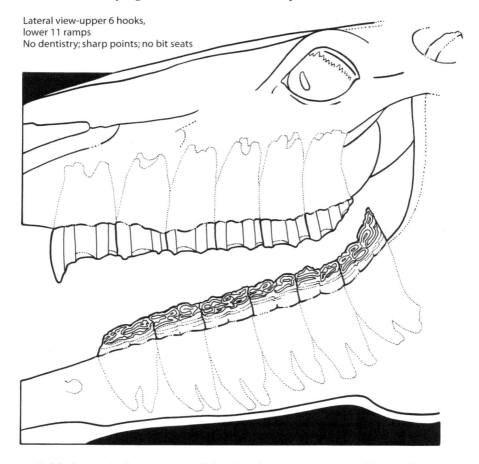

Lateral view-upper 6 hooks, lower 11 ramps
No dentistry; sharp points; no bit seats

Figure 5-32. Lateral view—upper 6 hooks, lower 11 ramps. No dentistry; sharp points; no bit seats.

Lower 6 Ramps

Elongation of the rostral border of the lower 6s (306, 406) is commonly called a *lower 6 ramp*. Like upper 6 hooks, lower 6 ramps develop when the rostral border of the lower 6 is located further forward than that of the corresponding upper 6. A ramp forms when the lower 6 is not worn evenly by its opposing tooth, resulting in vertical elongation of the rostral border of the lower 6 (see Figs. 5-37 and 5-42).

I find this malocclusion most often in gaited horses (Tennessee walking horses, Missouri foxtrotters, Standardbreds) and in miniature horses, but it can be found in any breed. In severe cases, the ramp may extend as far as the maxilla, damaging the mucosa of the gum or palate, and possibly even the bone.

Sharp Enamel Points

The prevalence and importance of sharp enamel points on the cheek teeth has long been appreciated. In 1906, Dr. Louis A. Merillat wrote, "Cutting and floating enamel points is the principal work of the animal dentist."[1] In my practice, almost all of the patients I see need some type of dental work in addition to removal of sharp enamel points. However, Dr. Merillat's point is well taken: sharp enamel points are a very common problem in the equine mouth, even in those that received thorough dentistry in the past 3 to 12 months.

Buccal Ulceration

Although sharp enamel points may be found in the mouths of healthy horses whose sole dietary intake is from grazing, there is no doubt these points are a source of discomfort to the horse when ulcerated areas are found in the adjacent buccal mucosa (see Fig. 1-6, Color Plates 37 and 39). Buccal ulcerations presumably cause discomfort when the horse is eating, but pressure from the bit or from the cheek pieces or noseband of the bridle can also cause discomfort during performance. Whether buccal ulcerations also present a health risk to the horse by allowing the systemic absorption of bacteria and/or their toxins from the oral cavity remains to be determined. In my opinion, the fact that sharp enamel points can cause discomfort to the horse is reason enough to diligently remove them.

I see an interesting effect of age on the prevalence of buccal ulceration associated with sharp enamel points. In my practice, well over 50% of horses between 3 months and 10 years of age have sharp enamel points on the upper arcades that are of such severity that the adjacent buccal mucosa is ulcerated. After 8 to 10 years of age, the incidence of buccal ulceration decreases, despite the fact that the size and sharpness of the enamel points appear to be the same in both age groups. In geriatric horses, whose teeth have depleted their reserve crown, sharp enamel points and subsequent buccal ulceration are far less common than in younger horses.

In my opinion, the presence of buccal ulceration indicates that *the horse needs dental care more frequently (or more thoroughly)* than it has had in the past. Some horses, particu- larly young horses, grind sharp points on their cheek teeth rapidly enough that ulcerations recur within 3 months of thorough dental care. In these horses the interval between dental examinations should be substantially less than the typical recommendation of every 6 to 12 months.

Retained Premolar Caps

Premolar caps refer to the deciduous teeth of the 6s, 7s, and 8s (Fig. 5-33). These deciduous premolars are normally shed as the permanent teeth erupt at around $2^{1}/_{2}$ years, 3 years, and $3^{1}/_{2}$ years of age, respectively (although these eruption times can vary by several months). Many of these caps show evidence of having harbored infection in the narrow space between the cap and the underlying permanent tooth: on removal, the underside of the cap is discolored and is covered by a malodorous exudate.

Presumably, bacteria gain entry to the space between deciduous and permanent tooth as soon as the junction between these teeth is exposed above the gingival margin. Because bacterial infection of this space could conceivably lead to gingival inflammation, I remove these caps as soon as the junction between deciduous and permanent tooth is apparent on visual examination of the mouth. I do not wait until the horse shows chewing, bitting, or other training problems.

Waves

Wave mouth is a common malocclusion (Fig. 5-34). It refers to an abnormal dorsal-ventral curvature of the molar table. Although wave mouth can originate in either an upper or a lower arcade, it is by far more common in the lowers. In such cases the teeth in the center of the lower arcade(s) are taller than normal, and the corresponding teeth in the upper arcade(s) are shorter than normal.

The most common configuration is an "8-high" wave, in which tall lower 7s, 8s, and 9s cause excessive wear of their opposing uppers. This wave formation is often found in horses in their midteens or older that have not had adequate dental care on a regular basis. Other wave formations are occasionally seen; in general, they include the 9s, regardless of which other teeth are involved.

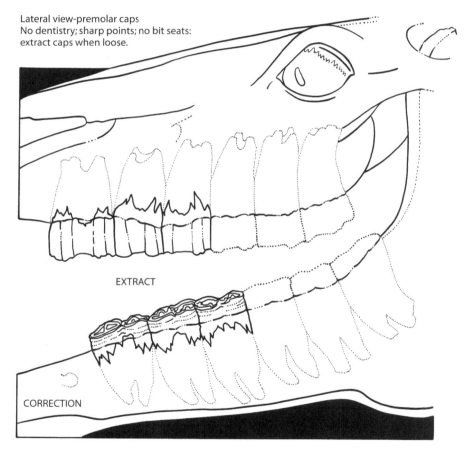

Lateral view-premolar caps
No dentistry; sharp points; no bit seats:
extract caps when loose.

EXTRACT

CORRECTION

Figure 5-33. Lateral view—premolar caps. No dentistry; sharp points; no bit seats: extract caps when loose. (This would never occur in a normal horse, all caps being ready at the same time, plus all molars present.)

The reason(s) waves develop is not known. It is theorized that they form because of a mortar-and-pestle effect of the dominating teeth on the opposing teeth during mastication. But why most waves involve the lowers dominating the uppers is not known. The upper cheek teeth are wider than the lowers, so it is possible that these wider teeth are slightly softer than the more compact lowers.

The upper 9 is a commonly overpowered tooth, probably because the 9s usually are the oldest teeth in the adult horse's mouth, having been the first permanent cheek teeth to erupt (at around 12 months of age). Thus they are the first to be worn past their enamel infoldings, making them less resistant to abrasion. If the upper cheek teeth are slightly softer than the lowers, then it stands to reason that the upper 9s are more easily overpowered by the lower 9s than the reverse situation (upper 9s overpowering the lower 9s) (Figs. 5-35 and 5-36).

Although the horse may be able to grind plant material efficiently enough with a wave mouth, I take a fairly aggressive approach to waves to preserve what remains of the teeth being overpowered. Reducing the height of the dominant teeth takes the overpowered and overworn teeth out of occlusion for a time, but it spares them further abrasion until crown height is restored (by eruption), and thus maximizes their useful lifespan. In geriatric horses with little or no reserve crown, this strategy simply delays expiration and loss of the overworn teeth; restoration of crown height generally does not occur because there is insufficient reserve crown.

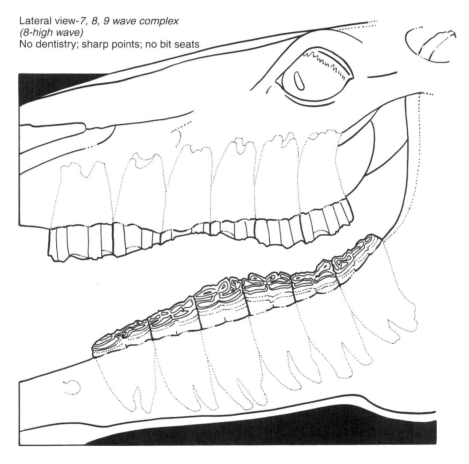

Figure 5-34. Lateral view—7, 8, 9 wave complex; (8-high wave). No dentistry; sharp points; no bit seats.

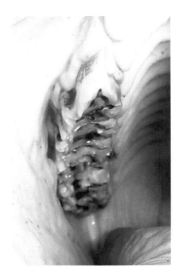

Figure 5-35. An example of cupped uppers in quadrant one.

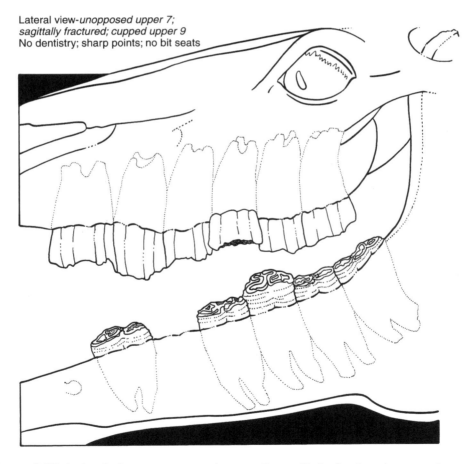

Figure 5-36. Lateral view—unopposed upper 7; sagittally fractured; cupped upper 9. No dentistry; sharp points; no bit seats.

Waves can begin in horses as young as 5 years of age, so thorough dental care should not be overlooked in young adult horses. The sooner a wave is reduced, the more the overpowered teeth are spared excessive wear. Reducing a wave when it is small also requires less removal of crown from the dominant teeth, ultimately prolonging the lifespan of those teeth, too. The longer a wave remains unresolved, the greater the wear on the overpowered teeth, the more extreme the wave becomes, and the more time and effort it takes to reduce the wave.

Another reason for treating waves aggressively is that they can limit rostral -caudal movement and even lateral excursion of the mandible, potentially impeding mastication and affecting athletic performance. Horses with severe wave mouth frequently have evidence of periodontal infection, which is yet another good reason for correcting waves as early as possible. (Periodontal disease is discussed in Chapter 7.)

Upper Wave Complex

An upper wave occurs when the upper 8 and 9, and possibly the 10, dominate the corre sponding lowers, resulting in pronounced ventral curvature of the upper arcade and a corresponding dip in the lower arcade. This condition is sometimes called a *reverse wave,* because the most common configuration of wave mouth is dorsal curvature of the lower arcades (Fig. 5-37).

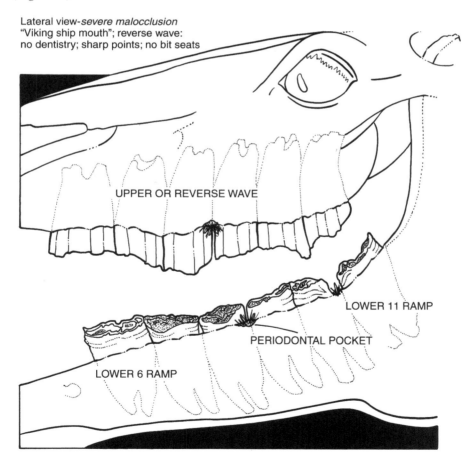

Figure 5-37. Lateral view—severe malocclusion, called "Viking ship mouth." Reverse wave: no dentistry; sharp points; no bit seats.

Upper wave complex is a relatively common problem in young racehorses and in mature horses if not corrected early. Two possible mechanisms for this particular configuration are disparity in eruption times between the uppers and lowers (allowing the uppers to dominate the lowers), especially involving the 9s, and the formation of excessive transverse ridges (see later discussion) on the upper 8s. This upper wave complex can interfere with mastication and performance by limiting rostral-caudal movement of the mandible.

"Impacted" Lower 10s

A similar malocclusion to the upper 8-9 wave complex occurs in young horses when the upper 10 dominates the lower 10. Owing to the curve of Spee (slight ventral curvature of the lower arcade), the lower 9s and 11s converge slightly, which can impede eruption of the lower 10 (Fig. 5-38). As a result, the upper 10 may elongate and dominate the lower 10. As with the upper 8-9 wave, this configuration can interfere with rostral-caudal movement of the mandible, and thus affect mastication and performance.

Excessive Transverse Ridges

Transverse ridges are found on the occlusal surfaces of the cheek teeth in most horses. The convoluted folds of enamel within the substance of the tooth that come into relief by wear of the surrounding, softer dentin form them. The relative height of the enamel ridges and the depth of the dentin valleys vary considerably from horse to horse, and even from tooth to tooth in the same horse.

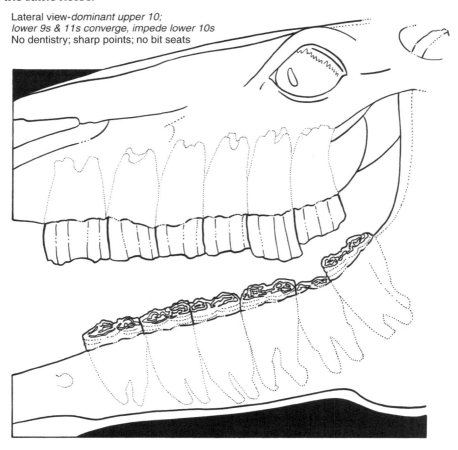

Lateral view-*dominant upper 10;*
lower 9s & 11s converge, impede lower 10s
No dentistry; sharp points; no bit seats

Figure 5-38. Lateral view—dominant upper 10; lower 9s and 11s converge, impede lower 10s. No dentistry; sharp points; no bit seats.

Although it is fairly common for the molar table to have a slight "washboard" appearance, these enamel ridges are usually only 2 to 3mm (1/8 inch) in height, from the depth of the valley to the tallest peak. Enamel ridges of greater height (excessive transverse ridges, or ETRs) can present a problem during mastication, because they may limit rostro-caudal movement of the mandible when the cheek teeth are in occlusion (Fig. 5-39).

In effect, ETRs may "entrench" the lower cheek teeth into a set path of movement across the uppers during the power stroke of mastication, which can contribute to abnormal wear. ETRs may also affect behavior or performance during ridden exercise by limiting rostral-caudal movement of the mandible as the horse flexes and extends its poll. In addition, they may contribute to upper wave formation in young horses, as discussed earlier.

Contributing Factors

The irregular surface of the molar tables is widely considered to be normal and even advantageous, because it provides a rough, abrasive surface for efficient grinding of plant material. The comparison is often made between the efficiency of a millstone with a smooth surface and one with a roughened surface.

Paradoxically, in my experience, transverse ridges tend to be far less pronounced (and may even be absent) in horses grazing very fibrous plant material, such as native grasses in many parts of the world. Evidently, the more fibrous or abrasive forages cause a greater amount of enamel wear, resulting in a smoother molar table.

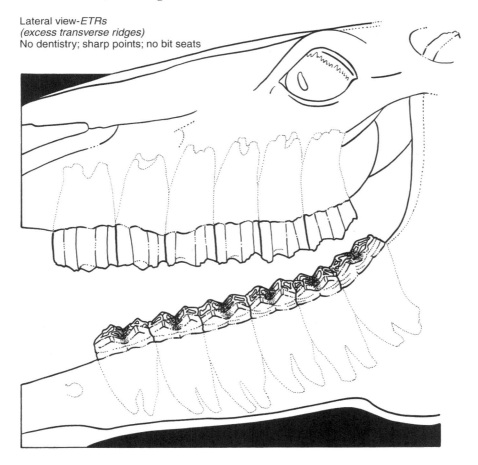

Lateral view-*ETRs*
(excess transverse ridges)
No dentistry; sharp points; no bit seats

Figure 5-39. Lateral view—ETRs (excessive transverse ridges). No dentistry; sharp points; no bit seats.

It could thus be speculated that ETRs are more likely to be found in horses on an "artificial" diet of hay and some type of concentrate. Another possible contributor to ETR formation is the relative hardness of the teeth. In my experience, ETRs are more likely to be found in horses that have rapidly recurring sharp enamel points, suggesting that the dentin is softer than normal in these teeth.

Cupping

Cupping of a molar refers to the formation of an abnormal concavity in its occlusal surface. Cupping occurs when the crown is worn past the level at which enamel is enfolded within the tooth's complex structure. Beyond this point the tooth is softer and less resistant to wear. As a result, the occlusal surface becomes concave, or cupped out, by the action of its opposing tooth (see Fig. 5-35 and Color Plate 42).

Cupping is most commonly seen in the uppers, possibly because these teeth are softer than the narrower, more compact lowers. The upper 9s are the oldest of the cheek teeth (having been the first permanent cheek teeth in wear), so they are the first to become excessively worn and cupped out. The upper 8s and 10s generally are the next to wear out.

Cupped-out teeth are nearing the end of their useful life. To preserve what reserve crown remains, a ration that requires minimal grinding should be recommended. Options include one of the "senior" rations (a complete feed that requires minimal grinding by the cheek teeth) or a pelleted feed made into a wet mash.

Steps

Abrupt changes in the height of the molar table are referred to as steps (Fig. 5-40). Typically they result from loss of part or all of a tooth, which allows the opposing tooth to become longer than its neighbors because it is no longer being worn at the same rate. Excessive wear (past the enamel infoldings) of the upper cheek teeth can also allow step formation, because excessively worn teeth are softer than normal.

Steps can cause the same kinds of problems as excessive transverse ridges (see p. 99), because they can "lock" the mandible into very limited rostral-caudal movement. If left uncorrected, an over long tooth can eventually invade the soft tissues and bone in the space left by the lost tooth. For these reasons, I treat steps fairly aggressively, sometimes reducing the height of the overlong tooth to below that of its neighbors if I will be unable to reexamine the horse within the next 3 to 6 months. Lowering the height of the overlong tooth to below the molar table does not interfere with masticatory efficiency, because this unopposed tooth does not actively participate in mastication.

Shear Mouth

Shear mouth refers to a dramatic increase in the molar table angle from the normal 12 to 15 degrees (Fig. 5-41). This abnormality results from a major and long-standing alteration in the direction of masticatory forces on the affected arcade. Dental pain is probably the most common cause of shear mouth. Loose or fractured cheek teeth cause the horse to alter the way it chews because of pain and/or displacement of the affected tooth. Over time, this pattern of mastication results in uneven wear of the cheek teeth on that side of the mouth.

In addition to an alteration in the molar table angle, the cheek teeth in both the upper and lower arcades on the affected side may be much longer than those on the opposite side of the mouth (the side doing the work of mastication). It is common to find a corresponding abnormality in the incisor line, such as wedge or slant mouth (see Fig. 5-31, p. 92) in these cases.

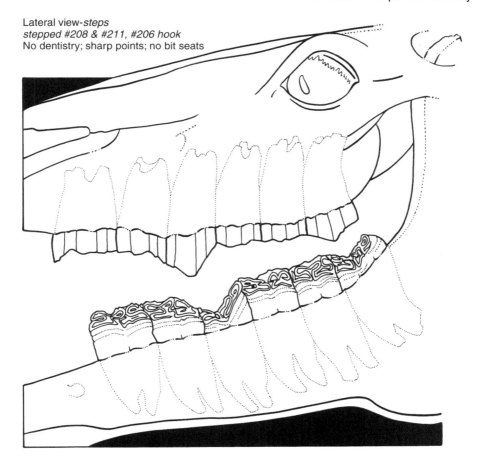

Lateral view-*steps*
stepped #208 & #211, #206 hook
No dentistry; sharp points; no bit seats

Figure 5-40. Lateral view—steps (stepped #208 and #211, #206 hook). No dentistry; sharp points; no bit seats.

Upper 11 Hooks and Lower 11 Ramps

Hooks and ramps can form on the caudal margin of the 11s (hooks on the upper 11s, ramps on the lower 11s) for the same reason they form on the 6s: uneven occlusion, and thus uneven wear (Fig. 5-42; see also Figs. 5-32 and 5-37). Hooks or ramps on the 11s can occur in conjunction with ramps or hooks on the 6s. For example, it is common to find lower 11 ramps and upper 6 hooks in the same mouth. This combination of abnormalities evidently indicates that the lower arcade is aligned a little caudal to the upper arcade.

Lower 11 ramps often become so long that they impinge on the roof of the mouth. This situation is potentially hazardous, because the palatine artery is located very close to this area. A common observation by owners or riders in such cases is that the horse resists any maneuver that necessitates poll flexion. Stopping is one such maneuver, so a common complaint is that the horse is difficult to stop. Correction of this malocclusion results in dramatic improvement in the horse's performance and attitude during work (Figs. 5-42 and 5-43).

Lateral view-shear mouth of 2nd and 3rd
quadrants; loose #309, overgrown #209
No dentistry; sharp points; no bit seats

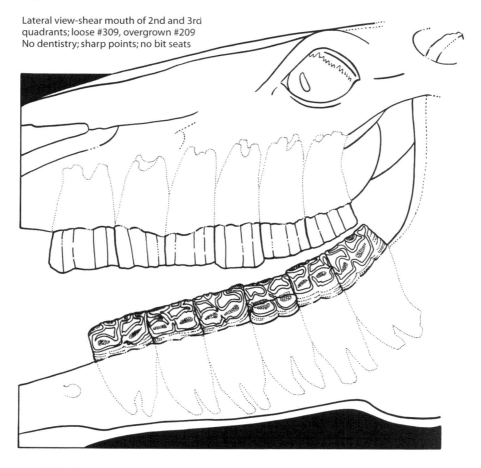

Figure 5-41. Lateral view—shear mouth of second and third quadrants; loose #309, overgrown #209. No dentistry; sharp points; no bit seats.

Importance of Bit Seats

Formation of a bit seat involves shaping the rostral occlusal margin of the first cheek tooth (the 6) to round its blocklike leading edge (Figs. 5-44 and 5-45). Although the squared rostral profile of the 6s is not an abnormality, there are two reasons for routinely forming a bit seat, both of which are aimed at benefiting the horse:

1. Improved comfort in horses that must wear a bit
2. Facilitated entry of long food particles into the molar tables

As stated by Dr. Merillat1 in 1906, "Dentistry must respect the horse's mouth as the 'seat of the bit' as well as the mechanism of mastication." When pressure is applied via the reins, the bit can compress the adjacent soft tissues of the lips or cheeks against the rostral margins of the 6s, potentially damaging these tissues. Rounding the rostral margins of the 6s gives the soft tissues a little extra room when the bit is applied, reducing this compressive effect. This may also prevent pressure on the tongue from the bit, as the bit can rest on the bit seats rather than sliding down the front of the 6s onto the tongue resting on the bars.

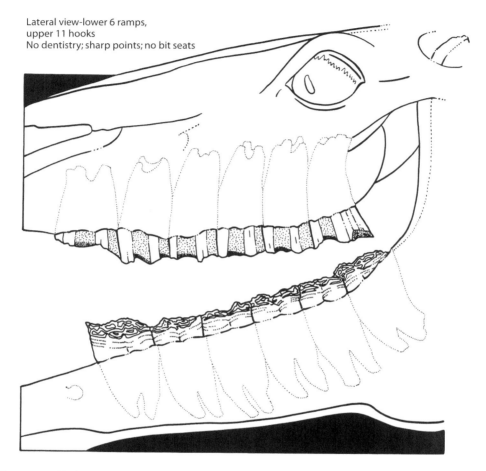

Lateral view-lower 6 ramps,
upper 11 hooks
No dentistry; sharp points; no bit seats

Figure 5-42. Lateral view—lower 6 ramps, upper 11 hooks. No dentistry; sharp points; no bit seats.

The second reason for forming a bit seat is more speculative. The premise is that rounding the rostral margins of the first cheek teeth removes a potential impediment to the entry of long stems of grass (or hay) into the molar tables: the blocklike edifices of the 6s. Forming a bit seat is described and illustrated in Chapter 6.

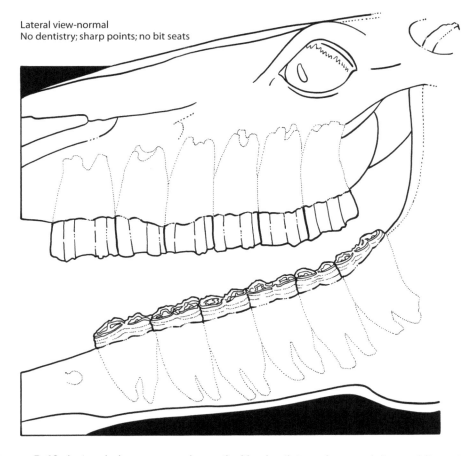

Lateral view-normal
No dentistry; sharp points; no bit seats

Figure 5-43. Lateral view—normal mouth. No dentistry; sharp points; no bit seats.

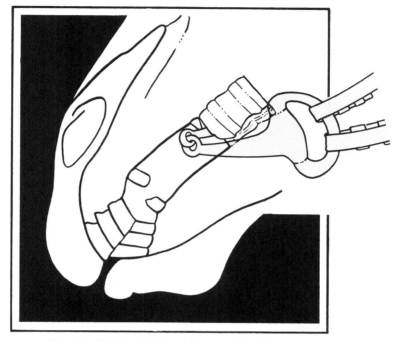

Bit against first cheek teeth; no bit seats, wolf teeth

Figure 5-44. Bit against first cheek teeth; no bit seats, wolf teeth present.

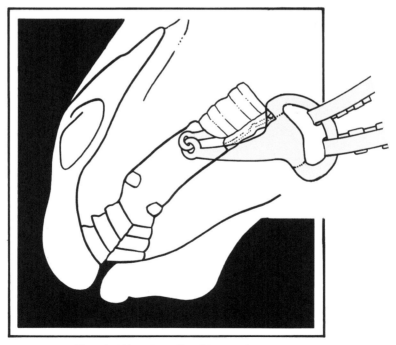

Bit against bit seats, wolf teeth removed

Figure 5-45. Bit against bit seats, wolf teeth removed, canines buffed.

REFERENCE

1.   Merillat LA: Animal dentistry and diseases of the mouth. In Veterinary surgery, Chicago, 1906, Alexander Eger.

*These assessments are described in Chapter 4.

CHAPTER 6

Routine Procedures

Tom Allen, Dale Jeffrey, Lawrence A. Moriarity

PRELIMINARY COMMENTS

Before beginning any dental procedures ensure that the patient is in a safe area and is adequately restrained. Set up your equipment for safety and work efficiency. Also make sure the owner knows what to expect, both procedurally and financially.

Order of the Procedure

Develop a routine that makes sense to you, allowing you to work systematically and efficiently (Figs. 6-1 and 6-2). The order I have found most efficient is to begin with the canines, work back along the molar arcades, then finish with the incisors. The incisors are worked on last because decisions regarding incisor reduction (the need for reduction, the amount to be reduced, etc.) should not be made until work on the molar arcades is completed.

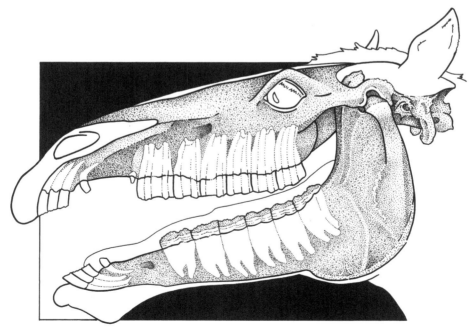

Figure 6-1. Lateral view. This is an excellent illustration of the location of the problems the equine dental practitioner has to evaluate and correct. Unfortunately practitioners do not have such an unimpeded view in their live patients.

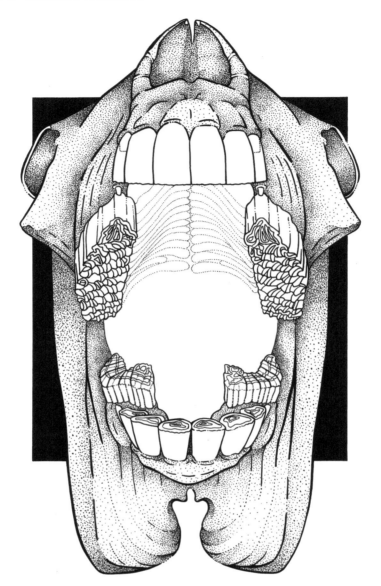

Figure 6-2. Rostro-caudal view. This is close to the view that practitioners have but lips, cheeks, and tongue and movement of the patient tend to obscure it, making a thorough recall of the structural relationships necessary.

Even if it is evident from the initial examination that incisor reduction is indicated, the degree of reduction needed will depend on what is done to the molar arcades. What may seem an adequate amount of incisor reduction if performed at the start of the procedure may prove to be inadequate or excessive, depending on how much the molar height has been changed to maximize molar occlusion.

There are two situations in which I vary this routine (Figs. 6-3 and 6-4):

1. Gross abnormalities of the incisors that make fitting the full-mouth speculum difficult or likely to place excessive pressure on some of the incisors or uneven load on the TMJs. Examples include severe wedge or slant mouth and severely malaligned permanent or deciduous incisors (Color Plate 43).

2. Problems that are likely to cause the horse greater discomfort if the mouth is held open for

any length of time. Examples include very sharp enamel points on the buccal margins of the upper cheek teeth or a fractured upper molar of which the buccal fragment protrudes laterally. In either instance, opening the mouth maximally with the speculum compresses the buccal mucosa against the sharp enamel points or tooth fragment, causing further pain and mucosal damage.

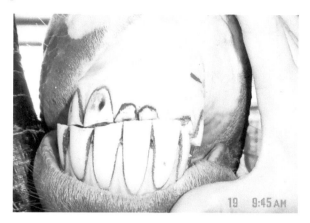

Figure 6-3. Gross abnormalities of incisors may necessitate addressing incisors before placement of speculum.

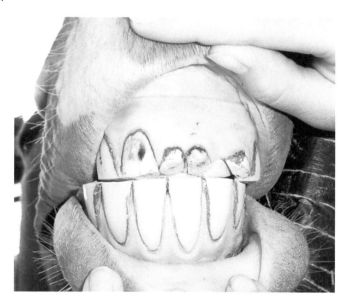

Figure 6-4. After the gross abnormalities of the incisors are corrected, the speculum can be positioned without causing excessive pressure.

In the first situation, I perform some incisor correction or extraction before proceeding with my usual routine. In the second situation, I reduce the sharp enamel points or remove the fractured fragments as the first order of business.

Working "Blind" Versus Working by Sight

Working "blind" means working without the benefit of seeing what you are doing as you are doing it; in other words, working by "feel" (Fig. 6-5). The advantage of working blind is that the horse need not be sedated and its head does not need to be elevated to any great degree.

Most practitioners who do not routinely sedate their patients work by feel, using hand floats. Although those who work by feel can periodically evaluate their progress by looking into the mouth, I like being able to see exactly what is happening as I work. Thus I perform almost all dental procedures by sight—that is, looking directly at the area being corrected. This approach requires a good light source, elevation of the patient's head (to minimize strain on the operator's back and legs), and good sedation (Fig. 6-6). I use a head-mounted light and support the patient's head in a dental frame (Color Plate 44).

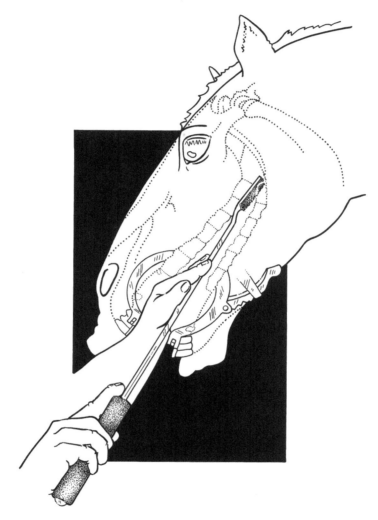

Figure 6-5. Working "blind" or by feel; better position for patient and practitioner.

Alternatively, a practitioner may work by sight while seated on a stool in front of the patient (Fig. 6-7). The advantage for the operator is less strain on the back and legs than when working standing. The advantage for the patient is the head need not be raised to the same height as when the operator works standing. Safety for patient and operator is paramount, so work seated *only when the patient is well restrained* in stocks or behind some other barrier (see Chapter 2).

Golden Rules

As with many aspects of equine practice, personal preference is an important determinant in how certain procedures are performed. What follows are descriptions of how I address the common dental problems described in the preceding chapter. These are my methods, developed over several years and many hundreds of horses, but they are just one way of achieving the desired goal of dental equilibration (Figs. 6-8 and 6-9).

I have two rules that guide my decisions when performing equine dentistry:

1. Never remove any part of any tooth unless doing so will help the horse (by improving comfort, masticatory efficiency, performance, and/or longevity).
2. Always remove any part of any tooth that is a hindrance to the horse.

These rules are easy to apply when the practitioner is familiar with the form and function of the various dental structures. However, what constitutes "enough" and "too much" may vary from one practitioner to another, depending on experience and on the individual patient's needs.

Other Guidelines

The following are some other guidelines for providing high-quality equine dental care:

1. Consider the patient's comfort, both as a goal of dental correction and during the procedure.
2. Tailor the treatment plan to the individual patient, taking into account your experience and equipment, the time available, the facilities, the owner's budget, the horse's temperament, and the potential for complications.
3. Do not hesitate to refer a patient to another practitioner if, for whatever reason, you feel you cannot provide the level of care required.
4. Don't let productivity interfere with the quality of your work; avoid scheduling so many horses on a given day that you don't do justice to any.
5. Enjoy your work!

Timed Breaks

An important practice I have adopted is to close the speculum and give the horse a short break every 10 minutes (see Fig. 2-7). I let the horse rest for about a minute while I massage its temporalis muscles. I then reopen the speculum and resume work. Although this strategy lengthens the overall time needed to complete the dental work on a particular horse, it improves patient comfort and thus cooperation.

This simple concession also reduces the severity of discomfort many horses experience for hours or days after major dental work. Because it is easy to get caught up in the work and lose track of time, I use a kitchen timer to alert me that 10 minutes have passed and I need to give the horse another break.

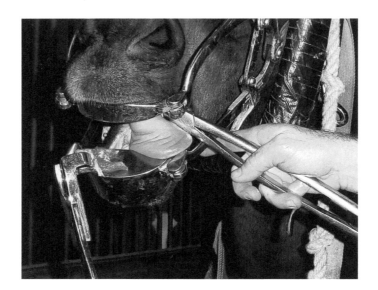

Color Plate 31. Stronger analgesic medications are used for major cheek tooth extractions.

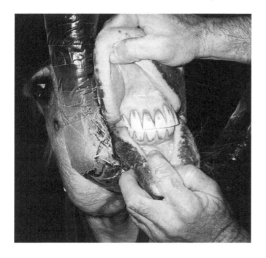

Color Plate 32. Inspection of incisors patient's chin in dental frame.

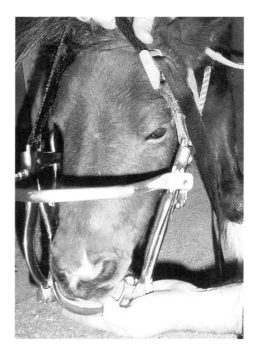

Color Plate 33. Applying the full-mouth with speculum.

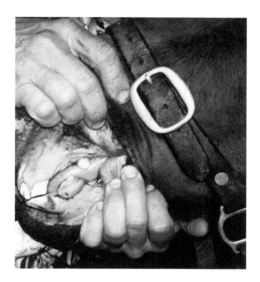

Color Plate 34. Massive tartar accumulation on lower canines.

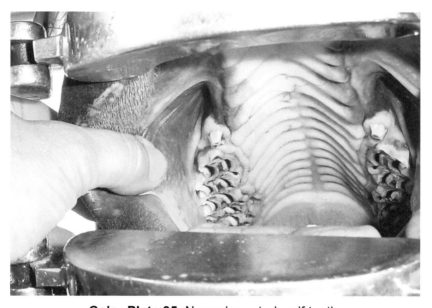

Color Plate 35. Normal erupted wolf teeth.

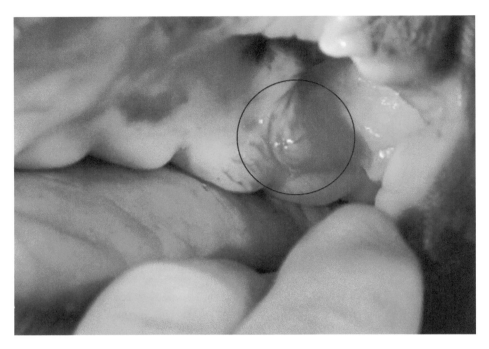

Color Plate 36. An unerupted wolf tooth covered with mucosa (the blood is from a lidocaine injection block). (*Courtesy World Wide Equine, Glenns Ferry, Idaho.*)

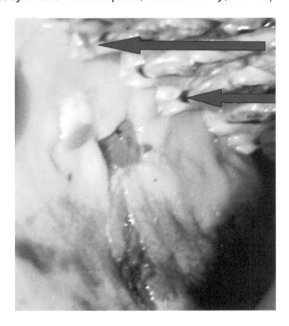

Color Plate 37. Buccal ulceration adjacent to the sharp points that caused it. (*Courtesy Tony Basile, El Dorado Hills. CA.*)

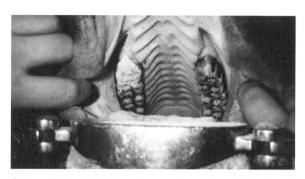

Color Plate 38. The 106 with a bit seat, the 206 without.

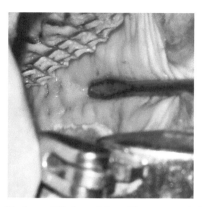

Color Plate 39. Sharp points with Resulting buccal ulcerations.
(*Courtesy Joe Allen, Edinboro, PA.*)

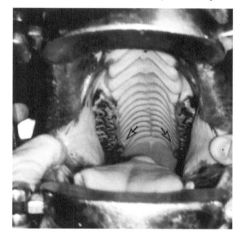

Color Plate 40. Sagittally fractured 109 and 209, the medial half is found tilting toward the palate.

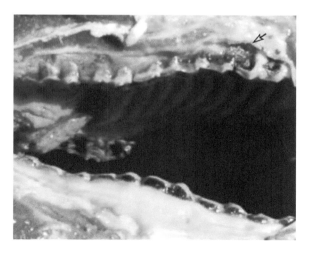

Color Plate 41. Periodontal pocket. (*Courtesy Tami Mitz, Brenhan, TX.*)

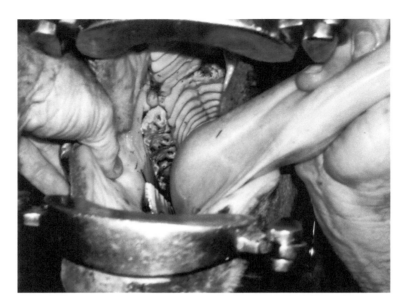

Color Plate 42. Example of cupped uppers in quadrant one and their relationship to the opposing quadrant four.

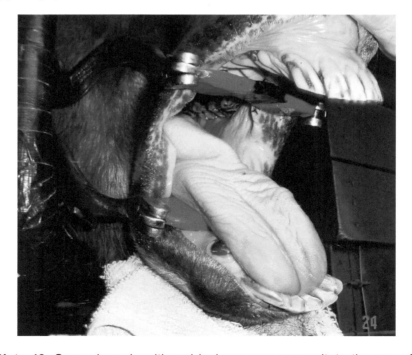

Color Plate 43. Severely malpositioned incisors may necessitate the use of special "cowbars" in the full-mouth speculum. The incisors of this patient extended straight forward and were loose, making the use of regular bit plates too risky.

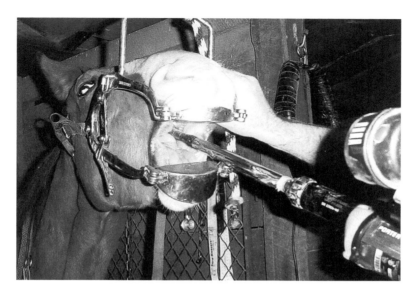

Color Plate 44. Working by sight.

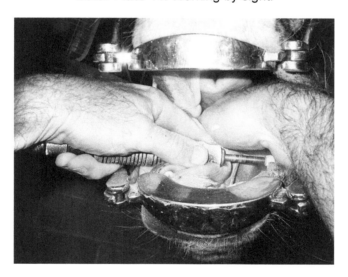

Color Plate 45. Spherical carbide burr being used on canines. When using this tool I protect the tongue and cheek by holding them out of the way with my other hand.

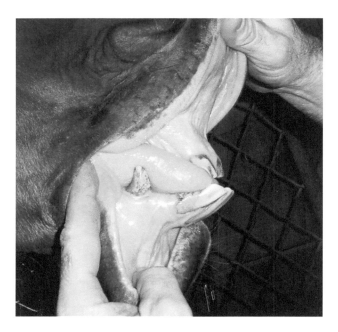

Color Plate 46. Massive tartar accumulation on canines and incisors.

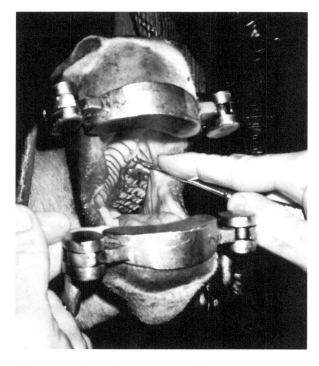

Color Plate 47. Elevation of gingival tissue around wolf tooth.

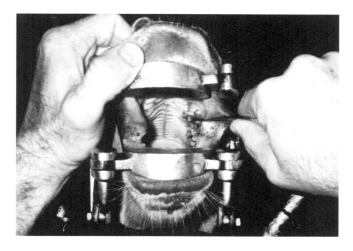

Color Plate 48. Application of deeper pressure to wolf tooth.

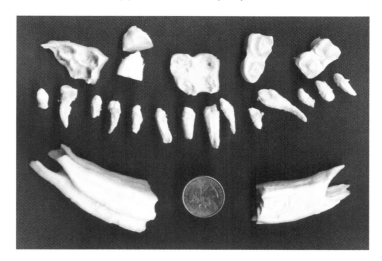

Color Plate 49. Assortment of teeth. *Top row*: upper 6 premolar cap; two incisor caps; three premolar caps. *Middle row*: assorted wolf teeth. *Bottom row*: molars.

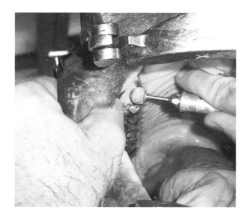

Color Plate 50. A, Forming an upper bit seat.

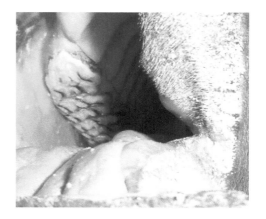

Color Plate 50. B, Final Result

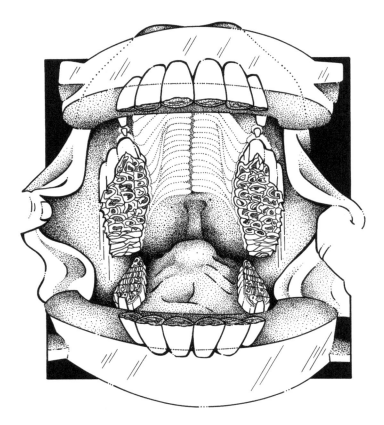

Figure 6-6. Working by sight allows visualization of more procedures, requires sedation and usually power equipment and a head support and light.

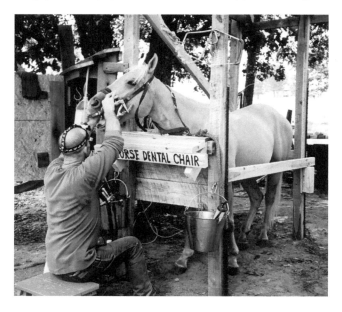

Figure 6-7. Working by sight while seated in front of the patient, horse's head is in a relatively normal position, yet practitioner is protected by barrier.

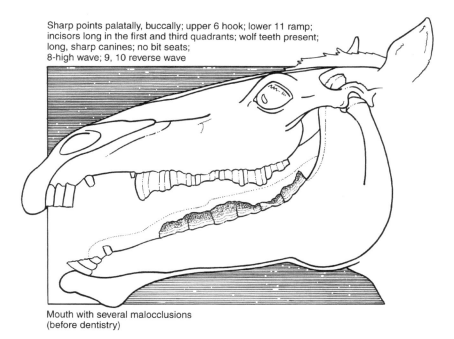

Sharp points palatally, buccally; upper 6 hook; lower 11 ramp;
incisors long in the first and third quadrants; wolf teeth present;
long, sharp canines; no bit seats;
8-high wave; 9, 10 reverse wave

Mouth with several malocclusions
(before dentistry)

Figure 6-8. Mouth with several malocclusions before dentistry. Sharp points palatally, buccally; upper 6 hook; lower 11 ramp; incisors long in the first and third quadrants; wolf teeth present; long, sharp canines; no bit seats; 8-high wave; 9, 10 reverse wave.

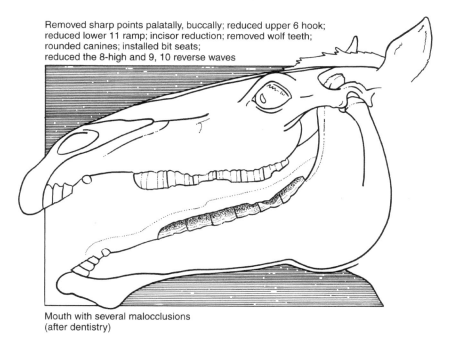

Removed sharp points palatally, buccally; reduced upper 6 hook;
reduced lower 11 ramp; incisor reduction; removed wolf teeth;
rounded canines; installed bit seats;
reduced the 8-high and 9, 10 reverse waves

Mouth with several malocclusions
(after dentistry)

Figure 6-9. Mouth with several malocclusions after dentistry. Removed sharp points palatally, buccally; reduced upper 6 hook; reduced lower 11 ramp; incisor reduction; removed wolf teeth; rounded canines; installed bit seats; reduced the 8-high and 9, 10 reverse waves.

Instruments

A wide variety of hand floats and motorized burrs, floats, and rotary disks is available (see Chapter 2). Selection of the most appropriate instrument for a particular task depends to some extent on practitioner preference. I currently use the PowerFloat* for almost all routine dentistry procedures involving floating. Other instruments I regularly use are described later in the relevant sections (Figs. 6-10 and 6-11).

A newly introduced instrument, the Horse Power Handpiece by World Wide Equine, offers similar advantages without the added weight of a drill. The unit is powered by a flexible cable shaft from a Dremel motor, with a foot pedal control available.

Previously, and even now periodically, I use one or both of the following tools for the majority of the procedures described in this chapter:

- 12-inch guarded motorized burr with vacuum attachment* (Fig. 6-12)
- Dremel handpiece with 1/2-inch spherical milled carbide burr (Color Plate 45, Figs. 6-13, 6-14)

A guard attachment is available for the Dremel tool handpiece. However, I prefer not to use a guard because mobile soft tissues such as the mucosa of the lip or cheek may become trapped between the guard and the high-speed burr. In these cases the guarded burr may cause more damage than would be caused by occasional abrasion from the unguarded burr. When using this tool I protect these tissues by holding them out of the way with my other hand.

NOTE: When using motorized equipment, keep the head of the instrument moving over the tooth to avoid overheating a particular area. It is also a wise precaution to wear eye protection of some sort.

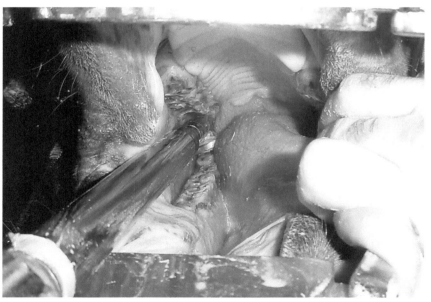

Figure 6-10. PowerFloat in use on 411 step.

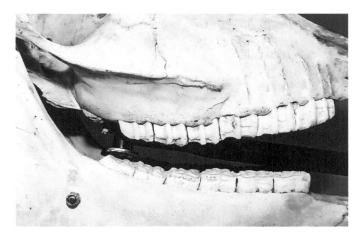

Figure 6-11. Another view of the PowerFloat reaching the 411. (*Courtesy D&B Equine Enterprises Inc., Alberta, Canada.*)

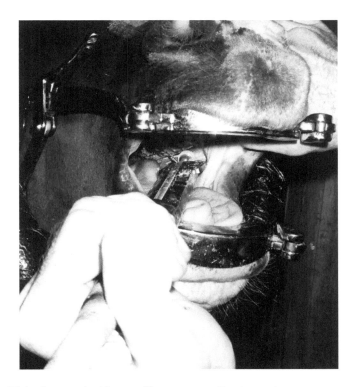

Figure 6-12. 12-inch guarded burr with vacuum attachment.

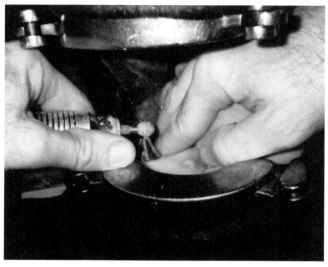

Figure 6-13. Canines being rounded.

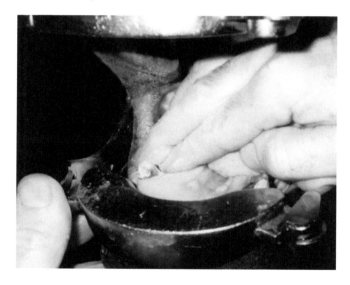

Figure 6-14. Rounded canines.

CANINES

Rounding Sharp Canines

Sharp canines can be blunted using a number of different tools, from hand floats to motorized instruments. I use the Dremel tool described above to remodel the canines. The tooth can be quickly and easily sculpted to the desired length and rounded shape in just a few seconds using this compact tool (see Fig. 6-13). Be sure to hold the tongue and lip out of the way with your other hand when sculpting the canines with motorized instruments.

It is not necessary—nor is it desirable—to reduce the height of the lower canines too much. If the horse subsequently begins "lolling" its tongue (hanging the tongue out the side of the mouth), the dental practitioner may be blamed for this habit, which is undesirable in a performance horse. The objective should simply be to blunt the canines so that they are unlikely to lacerate the horse's tongue or lips

In young horses with recently erupted canines, I may reduce the canines to just above the gum if I will not have an opportunity to reexamine the horse within the next 3 to 6 months. Recently erupted canines grow rapidly and may be long and sharp enough to be a problem again in just a few months. When performing this procedure, I make sure the crown of the tooth is well rounded and there are no sharp edges (see Fig. 6-14).

NOTE: Using canine cutters to crack off the top of a sharp canine tooth carries an unacceptably high risk of fracturing the tooth. I do not recommend this procedure when so many simpler and safer alternatives are available.

Erupting Canines

Erupting canine teeth can be a source of discomfort to the young horse as the overlying gingiva is stretched by the erupting tooth. In horses that must wear a bit, it may benefit the horse to hasten eruption by creating a defect in the gingiva overlying the erupting canine(s). Although the mucosa can be incised using a scalpel, a motorized burr can be used in sedated patients.

The burr is lightly touched to the gingiva for a second or two (at most), until a defect of about 3mm^2 is created and the tool sound changes, indicating that the burr has reached the underlying tooth. The advantage of using the burr is that a burred gingival defect bleeds less and is less likely to trap food particles than an incision made with a scalpel. In either case the underlying canine tooth generally erupts in a few days, without causing further irritation to the horse.

NOTE: Whenever the gingiva is invaded during dental work, *always check on the horse's tetanus immunization status* and recommend vaccination or booster if there is any doubt that the horse is adequately protected.

Tartar

Tartar is often found on the lower canines of mature horses; sometimes the accumulations can be several millimeters thick (Color Plate 46). Tartar can be quickly and easily removed using a motorized burr, wolf tooth forceps, or a dental elevator. The gingiva surrounding the tooth will likely bleed a little, because tartar accumulation typically causes gingivitis (see Chapter 7).

WOLF TEETH

In horses that must wear a bit, I routinely remove wolf teeth whenever I find them, because the potential for wolf teeth to cause discomfort in these horses far outweighs their usefulness to the horse. There are several methods for removing wolf teeth; mine is but one. The equipment I use consists of the following:
- Lidocaine (total of 3ml for a pair of wolf teeth)
- Wolf tooth elevator
- Wolf tooth forceps

Wolf tooth elevator sets that include elevators of various shapes and sizes are handy additions to the basic dental equipment inventory. Whichever instruments you use, be sure to keep them sharp or replace them when they no longer hold their edge. The wolf tooth elevator I use most often is scoop-shaped, with a head approximately 1cm (^{3}/$_8$ inch) wide. It was made by shortening an 18- to 25-cm (7- to 10-inch) half moon wolf tooth elevator[*] (Color Plates 47 and 48; Fig. 6-15).

The procedure is performed as follows:
1. Inject 1.5ml of lidocaine into the gingiva around each wolf tooth, whether normal or blind, a few minutes before extraction. (I proceed with other dental work while waiting for the lidocaine to desensitize the gingiva and periodontal tissues.)
2. Using the wolf tooth elevator, separate the gingiva and periodontal ligament from the tooth, being sure to work the instrument below the gingival margin around the entire circumference of the tooth. (After loosening the attachments to the tooth, I leave the wolf

teeth and work on another part of the mouth for a few minutes.)
2a. For blind wolf teeth, incise the gingiva at the rostral edge of the tooth using the wolf tooth elevator, then work the elevator between the tooth and the bone to loosen the tooth.
3. Remove the wolf tooth with the forceps. (Having loosened the tooth in Step 2 and left it alone for a couple of minutes, most wolf teeth are easily removed with a pair of forceps) (Color Plate 49).

NOTE: Whenever the gingiva is invaded during dental work, *always check on the horse's tetanus immunization status* and recommend vaccination or booster if there is any doubt that the horse is adequately protected.

FORMING BIT SEATS

Forming a bit seat basically involves rounding the rostral margin of the 6s. A variety of tools may be used, from hand floats to motorized instruments, depending on the practitioner's preference. I use the Dremel tool described earlier. Because I operate this burr without a guard, I use my other hand to protect the tongue and buccal mucosa from injury (Fig. 6-16).

I round the rostral edge of each 6, beginning just above the gingiva and ending on the rostral one third to one fourth of the occlusal surface. (As a guide, I sculpt to a distance on the occlusal surface approximately equal to the height of the exposed crown.) Using the Dremel tool, it takes only a minute or two to complete bit seats on all four teeth (Color Plate 50, Fig. 6-17).

CHEEK TEETH

Although work on the cheek teeth involves correcting abnormalities of individual teeth or groups of teeth, the ultimate objective is to balance all four molar arcades: normalize the height and angle of the molar tables as much as possible to maximize the comfort, masticatory efficiency, performance, and longevity of the patient. Following are descriptions of procedures for correcting specific abnormalities.

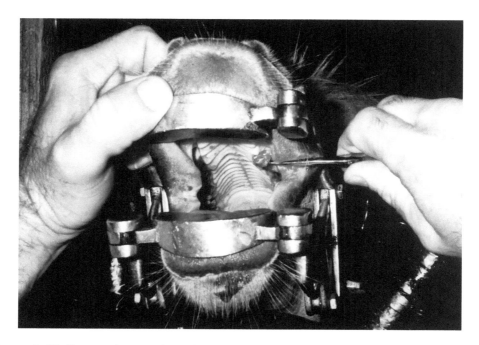

Figure 6-15. Eventual extraction of wolf teeth with elevator or with forceps.

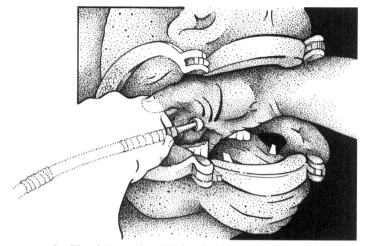

Small hand piece with carbide burr for bit seats or canines

Figure 6-16. Small hand piece with carbide burr for bit seats or canines. Use the other hand to protect soft tissue while forming bit seats.

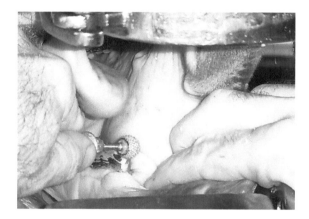

Figure 6-17. A, Forming lower bit seats.

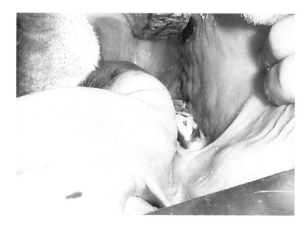

Figure 6-17. B, Final Results

Removing Sharp Enamel Points

Sharp enamel points can be removed using a variety of hand floats or motorized instruments (Figs. 6-18 to 6-20). Regardless of which instrument is used, the approach is the same. Because these sharp enamel points do not protrude beyond the occlusal surface (see Chapter 4), the objective is simply to *round the acute angle* between the occlusal plane and the vertical plane of the tooth.

It is important to remove as little tooth as possible from the occlusal surface. For this reason, I recommend keeping the float blade at an angle of approximately 45 degrees, rather than horizontal. For the upper arcades, the float blade is higher on the buccal side; and for the lower arcades the blade is lower on the lingual side (Figs. 6-21 and 6-22). With this approach an equal amount of tooth is removed from the occlusal surface as from the vertical face of the tooth, which is ideal. *Remove only that part of the tooth that is causing a problem to the patient.*

Keeping the float blade or motorized instrument horizontal, rather than angled, has the potential to remove too much of the occlusal surface. With aggressive technique, it is possible to inadvertently alter the plane of the molar table and even shorten the crown height at the buccal (uppers) or lingual (lowers) margin of the tooth (Fig. 6-23).

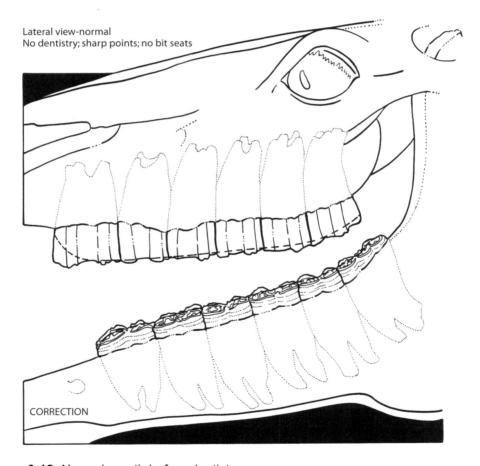

Lateral view-normal
No dentistry; sharp points; no bit seats

CORRECTION

Figure 6-18. Normal mouth before dentistry.

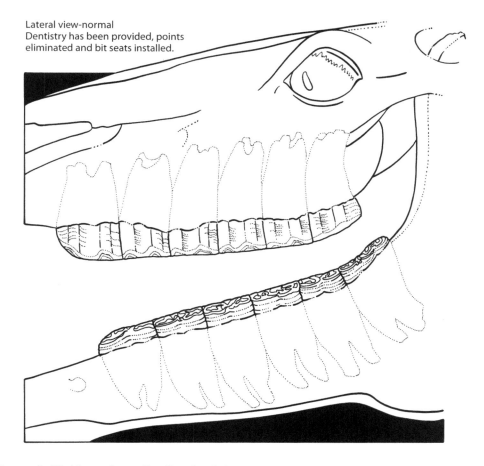

Lateral view-normal
Dentistry has been provided, points
eliminated and bit seats installed.

Figure 6-19. Normal mouth after dentistry.

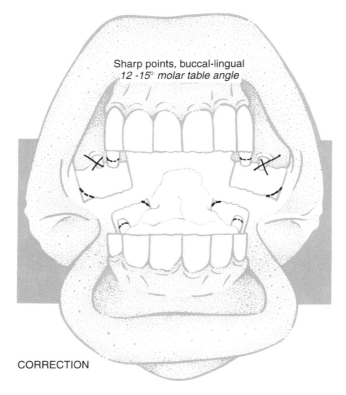

Figure 6-20. Removal of sharp enamel points. Sharp points, buccal-lingual 12 to 15 degrees molar table angle.

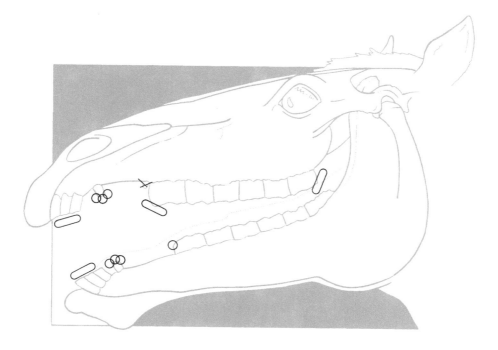

Figure 6-21. Position of instruments for various procedures, lateral view.

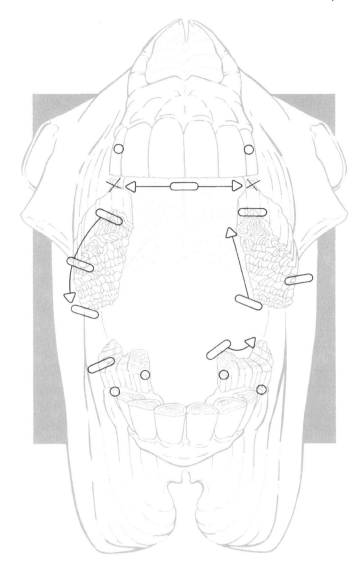

Figure 6-22. Position of instruments for various procedures, rostro-caudal view.

"Performance floats" can also negatively affect the tooth. This procedure involves smoothing the buccal and lingual-palatal faces of the tooth. Although it may delay the recurrence of sharp enamel points, in my opinion this aggressive approach removes too much tooth material, potentially weakening the tooth and shortening its functional life.

Checking Your Work

Using a full-mouth speculum, the enamel points are easily removed from the buccal margins of the first four upper cheek teeth and from the lingual margins of all lower cheek teeth in most patients (Figs. 6-24 and 6-25). However, access to the buccal aspects of the upper 10s and 11s can be a challenge. Nevertheless, it is important that sharp enamel points on these caudal teeth are not overlooked. I check the buccal margins of the upper 10s and 11s with my fingers to ensure that I have removed all of the sharp enamel edges. The lingual edges of the lower 10s and 11s should also be checked by palpation and reworked if necessary; this is another area that is often overlooked.

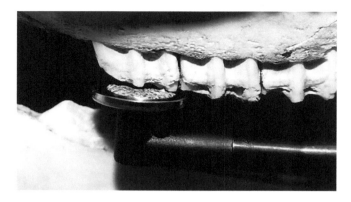

Figure 6-23. Positioning any instrument too near the occlusal table will remove excessive occlusal surface. (*Courtesy D&B Equine Enterprises Inc., Alberta, Canada.*)

An upturned (10- to 30-degree angle) slender-profile hand float* is a very useful tool for smoothing the buccal edges of the upper 10s and 11s. Because there is very little room to fit an instrument between the tooth and the cheek at this level, this slender float allows me to work on the buccal aspects of these caudal teeth without causing discomfort to the patient (see Figs. 2-2 and 6-5). A straight (i.e., not angled) float is best for doing touch-up work on the lower 10s and 11s.

Removing Premolar Caps and Remnants

Fragments of caps are often discovered when examining the cheek teeth, even in mature horses (see Fig. 5-32 and Color Plate 51). In most cases, caps are easily dislodged and removed with cap forceps (with or without a dental elevator). The cap is grasped with the forceps and removed by gently twisting the cap (Color Plate 52).

A small amount of bleeding often accompanies cap extraction, even when no obvious gingival tearing occurs. When part of the deciduous tooth clearly extends below the gingiva, it is best to elevate the gingival tissue from the buccal and lingual borders of the cap before extraction. Doing so prevents avulsion of the gingiva and additional hemorrhage. A long, sharpened screwdriver works well as an elevator for this and for prying loose caps off.

When removing caps from the upper cheek teeth, I try to draw the cap in a palatal direction, to minimize the risk of damage to the palatine artery from a sharp spicule of deciduous remnant. (The palatine artery runs parallel to the molar arcade, close to the palatal margins of the upper cheek teeth.) Although the potential for palatine artery damage is slight, this precaution seems worthwhile to me (Color Plate 53).

NOTE: Whenever the gingiva is invaded during dental work, *always check on the horse's tetanus immunization status* and recommend vaccination or booster if there is any doubt that the horse is adequately protected.

Removing Upper 6 Hooks

Upper 6 hooks can be removed using a variety of tools, from hand floats to motorized instruments (Figs. 6-26 and 6-27). My preference for removing small to moderate hooks is the Dremel tool described earlier. Another instrument may be better for removing hooks larger than 3cm³, because it can take too long to remove that amount of tooth using the Dremel tool alone. The Dremel tool can, however, be used for refining and finishing once the bulk of the hook has been removed with another instrument.

Regardless of which instrument(s) is used, the goal is to reduce the overlong portion of the tooth to level with the molar table (Fig. 6-28). If a bit seat is to be formed, it can be created at the same time or once other molar work has been completed.

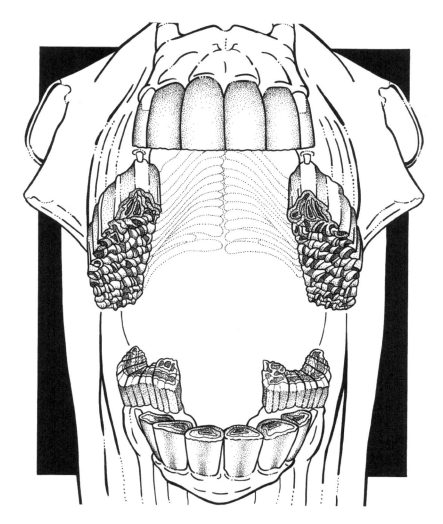

Rostro-caudal view, *before floating*

Figure 6-24. Before dentistry, rostro-caudal view (before floating).

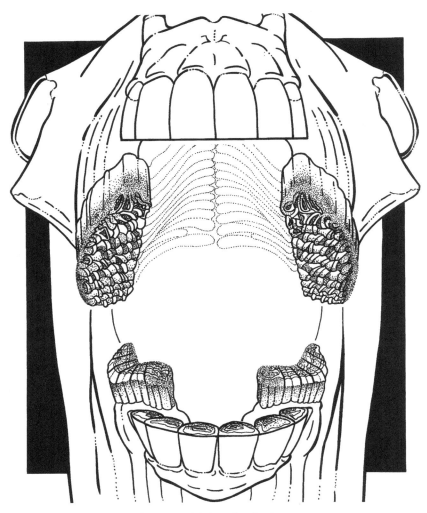

Rostro-caudal view, after floating

Figure 6-25. After dentistry, rostro-caudal view (after floating).

It is common for horses with upper 6 hooks to also have lower 11 ramps. Be sure to check for these ramps when upper 6 hooks are found. Reduction of lower 11 ramps is described later.

NOTE: When correcting severe or multiple abnormalities in one visit, give the horse a short break every 10 minutes by stopping work and closing the speculum for a minute.

Removing Lower 6 Ramps

As with upper 6 hooks, most lower 6 ramps are quickly and easily reduced with the Dremel tool described earlier (Figs. 6-29 to 6-31). Be sure to check for upper 11 hooks when lower 6 ramps are found. Reduction of upper 11 hooks is described later.

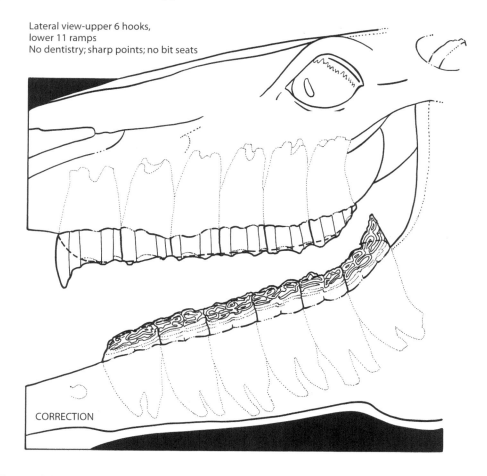

Lateral view-upper 6 hooks, lower 11 ramps
No dentistry; sharp points; no bit seats

CORRECTION

Figure 6-26 Lateral view of upper 6 hooks, lower 11 ramps.

Reducing Waves

Whether dealing with the typical 8-high lower wave or an upper wave complex (see Chapter 5), the goal is to remove the overlong portions of the dominant teeth (Figs. 6-32 and 6-33). Opinions among equine dental practitioners are divided on how much to reduce the overlong teeth. One opinion is to reduce the wave just enough to take the involved teeth out of occlusion until the next scheduled dental appointment. The rationale is that the overpowered teeth gain some respite but may still be able to participate in mastication if there is a gap of only a couple of millimeters between the dominant and overpowered teeth (Fig. 6-34).

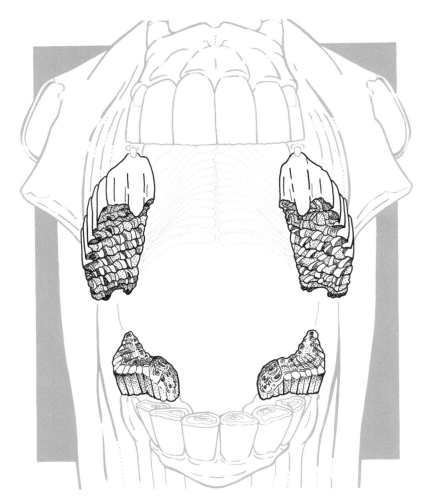

Rostro-caudal view, upper 6 hooks, lower 11 ramps

Figure 6-27. Rostro-caudal view, upper 6 hooks, lower 11 ramps.

My opinion is that it is best to normalize the molar tables as much as possible, as soon as possible. Although this strategy slightly reduces the surface area of the molar table available for mastication, it "unlocks" the restricted rostro-caudal movement of the mandible and eliminates any further wear on the overpowered teeth until they have erupted to level with the adjacent teeth (assuming they have sufficient reserve crown to do so). It is unlikely that this strategy significantly reduces masticatory efficiency; in fact, unlocking the mandible may improve overall masticatory efficiency by allowing the upper and lower arcades on both sides of the mouth to function optimally.

Waves can be reduced using a variety of tools, from hand floats to motorized instruments. My preference is the PowerFloat, although the long, guarded burr described earlier also makes short work of wave reductions. The new Horse Power Handpiece by World Wide Equine offers an advantage due to less weight required to be handled.

NOTE: When correcting severe or multiple abnormalities in one visit, give the horse a short break every 10 minutes by stopping work and closing the speculum for a minute.

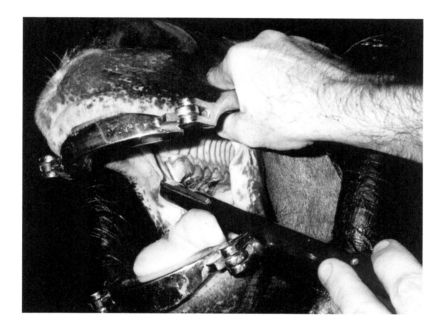

Figure 6-28. Addressing a 106 hook.

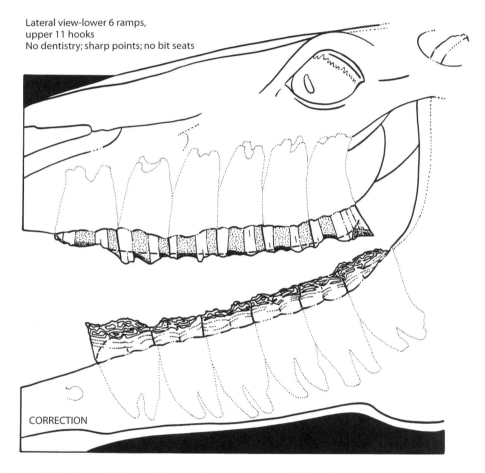

Lateral view-lower 6 ramps,
upper 11 hooks
No dentistry; sharp points; no bit seats

CORRECTION

Figure 6-29. Lateral view of lower 6 ramps, upper 11 hooks.

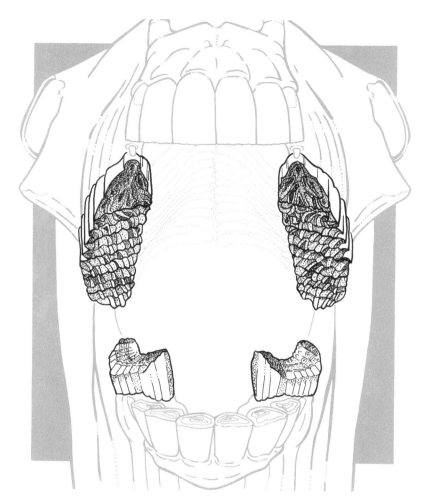

Rostro-caudal view, lower 6 ramps, upper 11 hooks

Figure 6-30. Rostro-caudal view, lower 6 ramps, upper 11 hooks.

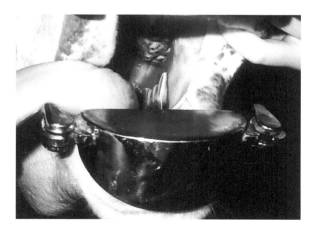

Figure 6-31. Lower 6 ramps (306).

Removing Excessive Transverse Ridges

Excessive transverse ridges can be removed with hand floats or with motorized instruments, such as the 12-inch guarded burr described earlier (Figs. 6-35 and 6-36). Remove only the prominent enamel ridges, and only those that appear to be hindering rostro-caudal movement of the mandible (Fig. 6-37). (These ridges are best evaluated by sighting along the molar table.)

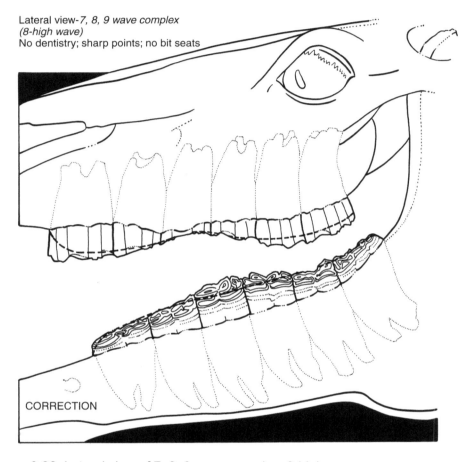

Lateral view-*7, 8, 9 wave complex*
(8-high wave)
No dentistry; sharp points; no bit seats

CORRECTION

Figure 6-32. Lateral view of 7, 8, 9 wave complex; 8-high wave.

It is not necessary—nor is it desirable—to remove all enamel prominences (i.e., smooth out the occlusal surface), especially on the 6s and 11s. Doing so can reduce the height of the crown, which shortens the functional life of the tooth and may even promote formation of a diastema (a gap between adjacent teeth), thereby increasing the potential for periodontitis to develop (see Chapter 7). To determine whether sufficient enamel has been removed, recheck rostro-caudal movement of the mandible (as described in Chapter 4) once all the dental work is completed.

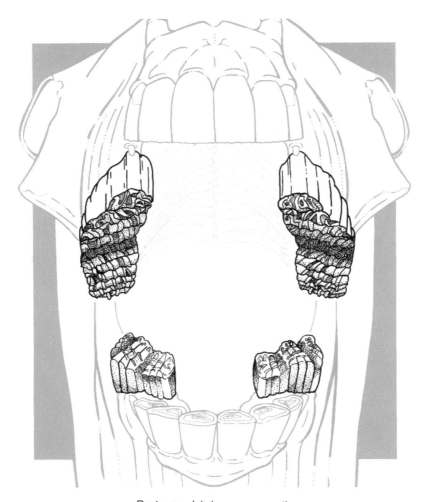

Rostro-caudal view, *wave mouth*

Figure 6-33. Rostro-caudal view, wave mouth.

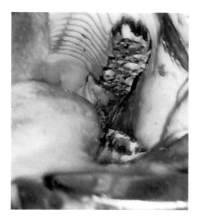

Figure 6-34. 8-high wave (7, 8, 9 involved).

Removing Steps

Steps may be reduced using a variety of tools, from hand tools to motorized instruments. Be sure to examine the opposing molar arcade carefully to determine the cause of step formation (e.g., lost, loose, or fractured opposing tooth) and correct any abnormalities accordingly (Figs. 6-38 and 6-39).

NOTE: When correcting severe or multiple abnormalities in one visit, give the horse a short break every 10 minutes by stopping work and closing the speculum for a minute (Fig. 6-40).

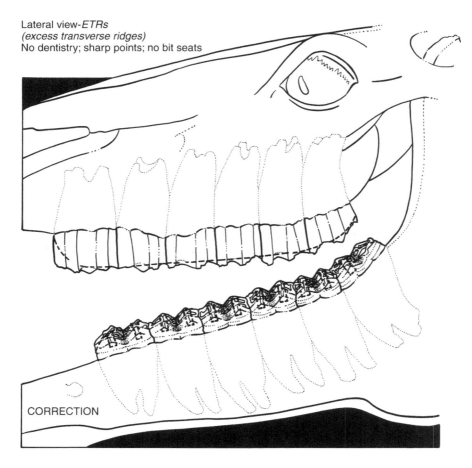

Lateral view-*ETRs*
(excess transverse ridges)
No dentistry; sharp points; no bit seats

CORRECTION

Figure 6-35. Lateral view of ETRs (excessive transverse ridges).

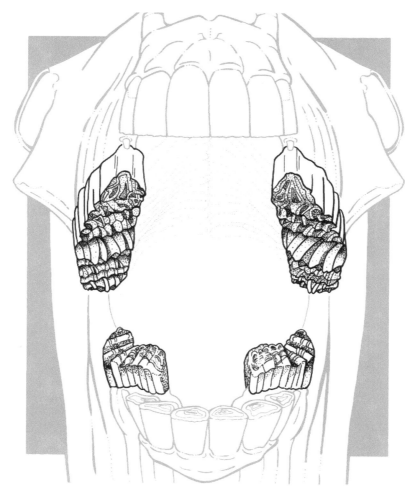

Rostro-caudal view, *ETRs*
(excessive transverse ridges)

Figure 6-36. Rostro-caudal view of ETRs.

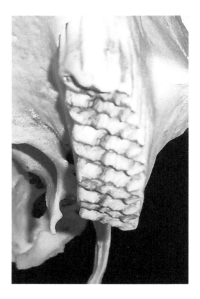

Figure 6-37. Example of ETRs, upper arcade.

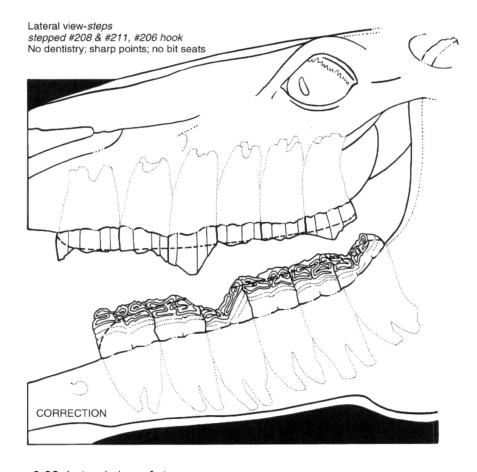

Lateral view-*steps*
stepped #208 & #211, #206 hook
No dentistry; sharp points; no bit seats

CORRECTION

Figure 6-38. Lateral view of steps.

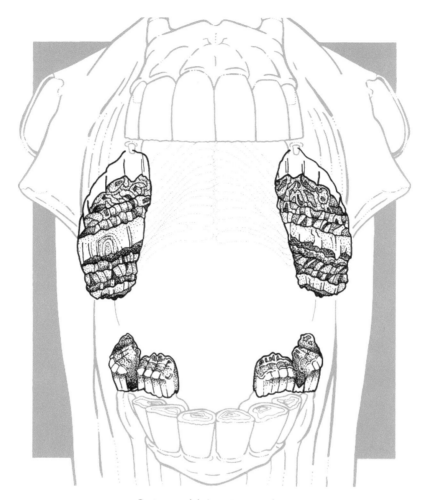

Rostro-caudal view, step mouth

Figure 6-39. Rostro-caudal view, step mouth.

Correcting Shear Mouth

The first step in correcting shear mouth is to identify and address the underlying cause (e.g., an infected, loose, or fractured tooth causing pain during mastication) (Figs. 6-41 to 6-43). The overlong portions of the affected cheek teeth are then reduced in height and the molar table angle is normalized using the instrument(s) of your choice.

Typically, reduction of molar height and restoration of the molar table angle involves removal of dental material from the buccal portion of the occlusal surface on the upper arcade and from the lingual portion of the occlusal surface on the lower arcade. Take care not to remove too much material (and thus excessively shorten the overall crown height), and be careful not to flatten the molar tables. There should be a 12- to 15-degree angle, sloping downward from palatal-lingual to buccal, when you are done (see Fig. 6-20).

NOTE: When correcting severe or multiple abnormalities in one visit, give the horse a short break every 10 minutes by stopping work and closing the speculum for a minute.

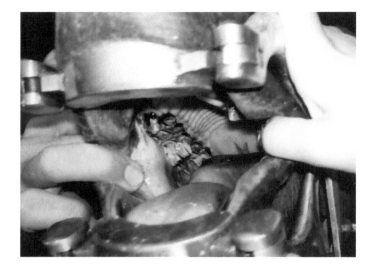

Figure 6-40. Steps.

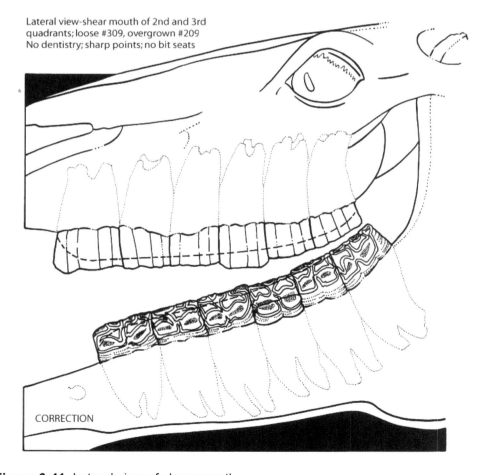

Lateral view-shear mouth of 2nd and 3rd
quadrants; loose #309, overgrown #209
No dentistry; sharp points; no bit seats

CORRECTION

Figure 6-41. Lateral view of shear mouth.

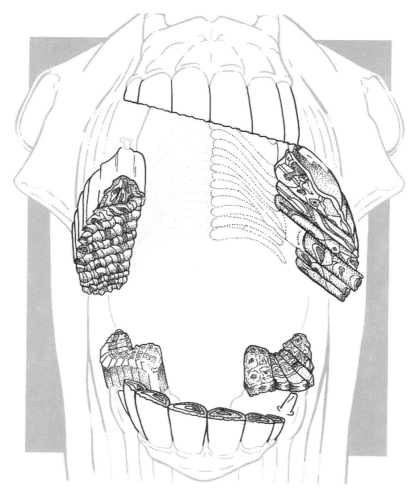

Rostro-caudal view, shear mouth

Figure 6-42. Rostro-caudal view of shear mouth.

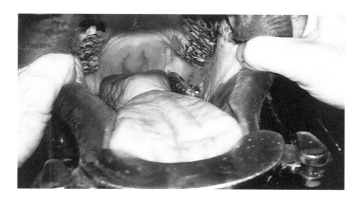

Figure 6-43. Shear Mouth.

Removing Lower 11 Ramps

Removing lower 11 ramps can be a challenge, because the close proximity of the buccal tissues, ramus of the mandible, and the base of the tongue hinders work on the caudal aspect of the lower 11s. I have yet to encounter a lower 11 ramp that I could not reduce with a motorized burr or float, or even a hand float. However, considerable patience and dexterity are often needed to work on these distant teeth. Care must also be taken to avoid traumatizing the adjacent tissues. After reducing the ramp, I use a hand float with an upturned carbide insert to remove any remaining sharp edges from the caudal aspect of the tooth.

Some equine dental practitioners keep molar cutters on hand for large lower 11 ramps that cannot be reduced using a float or burr. I have yet to encounter such a situation, so I do not recommend the purchase of molar cutters. Rather, if you encounter a malocclusion of any kind that you cannot reduce with the instruments you have on hand, I recommend referring the horse to another dental practitioner.

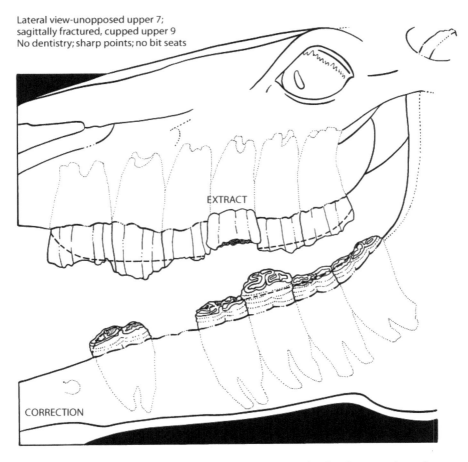

Figure 6-44. Lateral view; unopposed upper 7; sagittally fractured and cupped upper 9.

Removing Upper 11 Hooks

Upper 11 hooks can be removed with a variety of tools, from hand floats to motorized instruments. The caudal edge of the tooth may require finishing using the 30-degree upturned slimline float described for removal of sharp enamel points from the buccal margins of upper 10s and 11s (see Figs. 6-29 and 6-30).

Removing Fractured Cheek Teeth

Displaced fragments of fractured cheek teeth (most often the upper 9s) usually are easily removed with cap extractors or molar forceps (Figs. 6-44 to 6-48). Molar spreaders may be needed to loosen nondisplaced portions of the fractured tooth. (Not all molar fractures result in displacement of the fracture fragments; sometimes the fragments are held tightly in place by the neighboring teeth.) If the tooth has been damaged for some time, a step may have formed in the opposing arcade (e.g., overlong lower 9 with a fractured upper 9). The step should be reduced as described earlier. Peroral extractions are discussed further in Chapter 7.

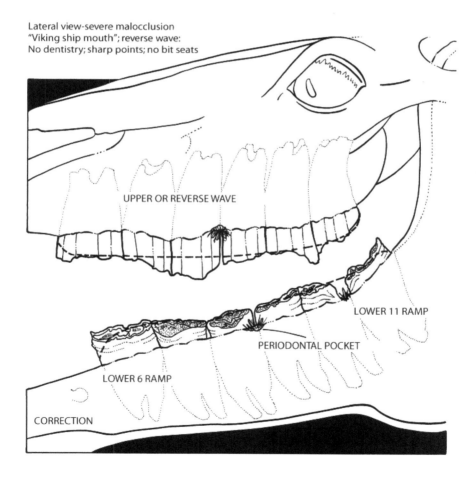

Figure 6-45. Laterial view; severe malocclusion (Viking ship mouth). Reverse wave.

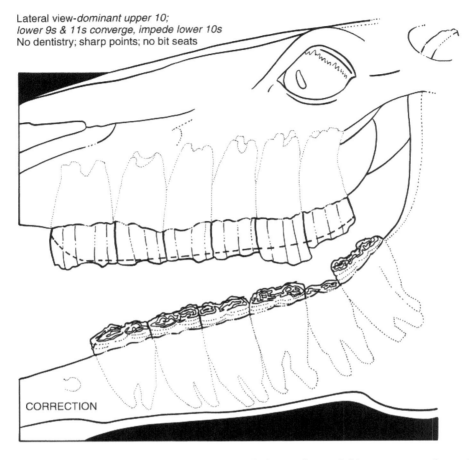

Lateral view-*dominant upper 10;*
lower 9s & 11s converge, impede lower 10s
No dentistry; sharp points; no bit seats

CORRECTION

Figure 6-46. Lateral view; dominant upper 10; lower 9s and 11s converge, impede lower 10s.

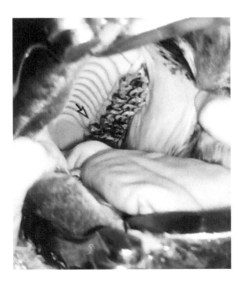

Figure 6-47. Palatally displaced fragment of sagittally fractured 209.

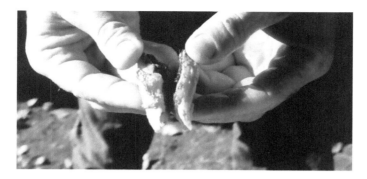

Figure 6-48. Extracted sagittally fractured 209.

INCISOR REDUCTION AND ALIGNMENT

Reevaluation of Molar Occlusion

Once work on the molar arcades is completed, I remove the speculum and repeat the lateral excursion test for molar occlusion (see Chapter 4, Figs. 4-11 through 4-15). In my opinion, if molar occlusion is less than 75%, some degree of incisor reduction is indicated to improve molar occlusion and maximize masticatory efficiency. Improving molar occlusion also extends the functional life of the cheek teeth, because the occlusal surfaces will wear more uniformly when molar occlusion is close to 100%. I recommend incisor reduction on the majority of mature horses when molar occlusion after molar work is less than 75%.

I do not routinely perform incisor reduction on horses less than 5 years of age, because their mouths are still adjusting to eruption of the permanent cheek teeth and loss of the deciduous premolars. In older horses that have undergone extensive dental correction for a severe malocclusion, and in which the degree of change is such that the horse may be uncomfortable while eating for a few days, I advise waiting until the next visit to perform incisor reduction (Fig. 6-49). Additionally, if molar occlusion is low, a mash made from a complete (senior type) pelleted feed is recommended.

Gags for Incisor Work

The full-mouth speculum must be removed for incisor work, because the bite plates prevent access to the occlusal surfaces of the incisors. There are a couple of options for keeping the patient's mouth open when working on the incisors. For quick procedures, the practitioner's hand can be placed in the interdental space. For more time-consuming procedures, or when both hands are needed, a wedge-type gag can be inserted between the cheek teeth (see Chapter 2).

I use a length of flexible plastic pipe and elastic cord to create a self-retaining gag. The diameter of the pipe used in a particular situation depends on the size of the patient, from 1½ inches for small patients to 3inches for large patients. The elastic cord is attached to each end of the pipe and runs around the horse's poll like the poll strap on a bridle (Fig. 6-50).

Incisor Table Angle Abnormalities

Before performing incisor reduction, consider the incisor table angle (see Chapter 4). If an overjet has increased the incisor table angle beyond the normal 10 to 15 degrees relative to the bars of the mouth, the table angle should be normalized. This procedure involves removing a small amount of tooth from the rostral (labial) part of the occlusal surface on the upper incisors and from the caudal (lingual) part of the occlusal surface on the lower incisors (Figs. 6-51 and 6-52).

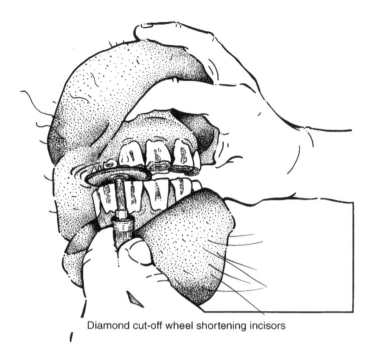

Diamond cut-off wheel shortening incisors

Figure 6-49. Diamond cut-off wheel shortening incisors. Reducing incisors.

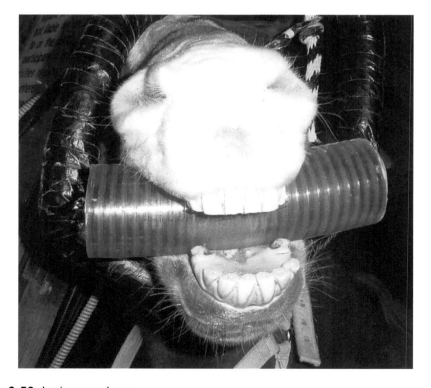

Figure 6-50. Incisor work gag.

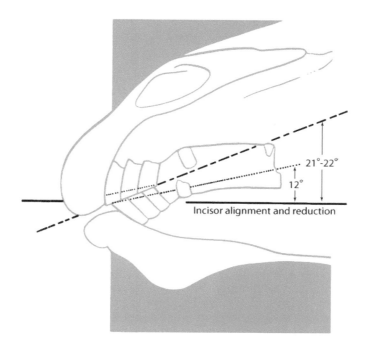

Figure 6-51. Incisor alignment and reduction. Incisor table angle correction.

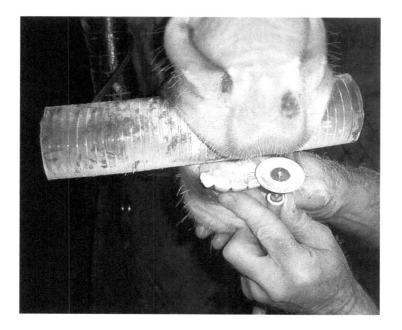

Figure 6-52. Incisor reduction in progress.

If an underjet has lowered the incisor table angle beyond normal, the table angle is corrected by lowering the rostral aspect of the occlusal surface on the lowers and the caudal aspect of the occlusal surface on the uppers.

In horses with severe incisor malocclusions, it may not be advisable (or even possible) to normalize the incisor table angle in one visit. In fact, it may never be possible to normalize the angle without invading the sensitive tissues of the incisors, which should be avoided.

Incisor Line Abnormalities

It is often advisable to correct abnormalities of the incisor line (wedge or slant mouth, smile, or frown; see Chapter 4) (Figs. 6-53 to 6-67). This procedure involves reducing the height of the incisors that protrude above or below the horizontal incisor line. For example, if the patient has wedge-slant mouth that is long in quadrants 1 and 3, the incisors in those quadrants should be reduced to level with the horizontal incisor line (see Fig. 6-54).

This procedure results in a gap at the lateral aspects of the incisor table, unless the incisors are so overgrown that all incisors in both arcades require reduction to restore normal incisor length and occlusion. In other words, if the incisors are so long that, after the wedge or slant, frown, or smile is corrected, the incisors need to be reduced even more to achieve good molar occlusion, then there will be no gap anywhere along the incisor line, because a new incisor line is created.

Incisor Reduction

Reduction of incisor height may be accomplished with hand floats or with motorized instruments such as burrs and diamond cut-off wheels. I use the flat side of a diamond cut-off wheel to remove excess crown and achieve the desired incisor length and table angle (Color Plate 54). Protective eyewear should be worn when using a cut-off wheel to reduce incisors. A mask should also be worn to avoid inhalation of airborne dental dust. A window fan directed in the appropriate direction helps by blowing the tooth dust away from the work area.

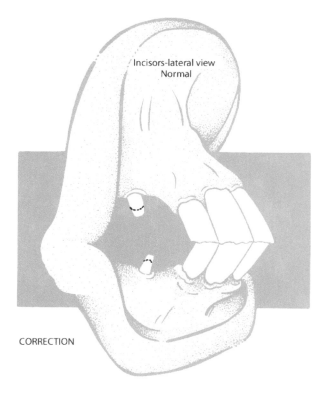

Incisors-lateral view
Normal

Figure 6-53. Lateral view of normal incisors.

CORRECTION

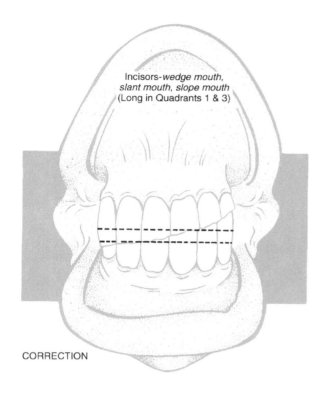

Figure 6-54. Anteroposterior (AP) view of incisors; wedge outh, slant mouth, slope mouth, diagonal mouth. Long in quadrants 1 and 3.

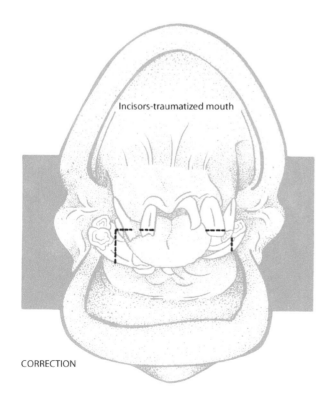

Figure 6-55. AP view of incisors; traumatized mouth.

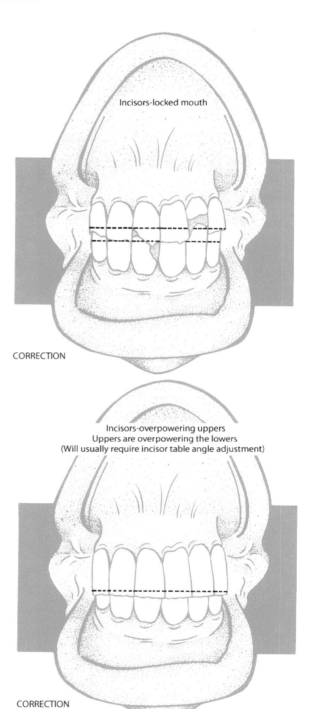

Figure 6-56. AP view of incisors; locked mouth.

Figure 6-57. AP view of incisors; overpowering uppers. Uppers are overpowering the lowers. Usually requires incisor table angle adjustment.

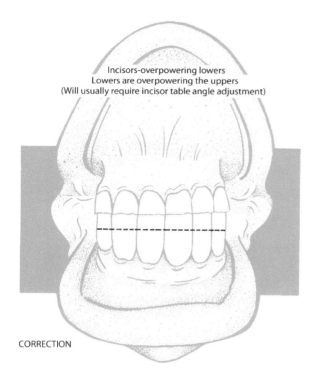

Incisors-overpowering lowers
Lowers are overpowering the uppers
(Will usually require incisor table angle adjustment)

CORRECTION

Figure 6-58. Incisors; overpowering lowers. Lowers are overpowering the uppers. Usually requires incisor table angle adjustment.

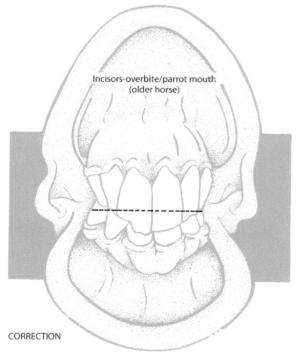

Incisors-overbite/parrot mouth
(older horse)

CORRECTION

Figure 6-59. AP view of incisors; overbite (parrot mouth) in an older horse. (Upper 6 hooks, lower 11 ramps often accompany overbite.)

Figure 6-60. Lateral view of incisors; overbite (parrot mouth) in an older horse. (Upper 6 hooks, lower 11 ramps often accompany overbite.)

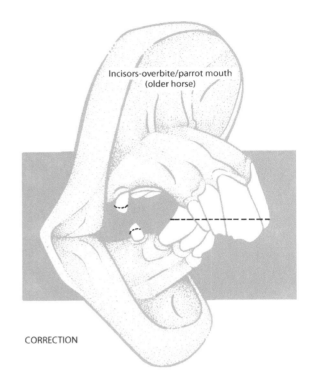

Incisors-overbite/parrot mouth
(older horse)

CORRECTION

Figure 6-61. Lateral view of incisors; overbite (parrot mouth) in a younger horse. (Upper 6 hooks, lower 11 ramps often accompany overbite.)

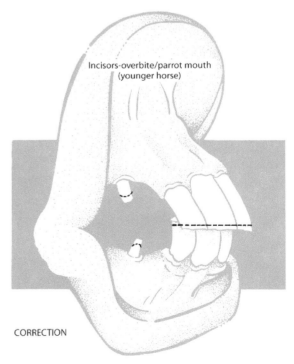

Incisors-overbite/parrot mouth
(younger horse)

CORRECTION

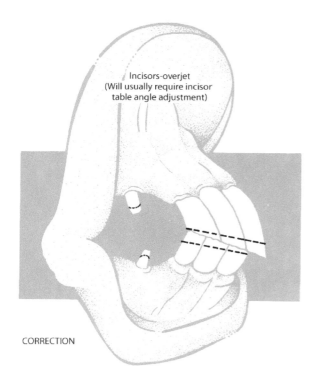

Incisors-overjet
(Will usually require incisor
table angle adjustment)

CORRECTION

Figure 6-62. Lateral view of incisors; overjet. Usually requires incisor table adjustment.

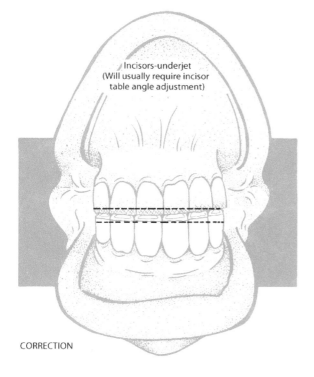

Incisors-underjet
(Will usually require incisor
table angle adjustment)

CORRECTION

Figure 6-63. AP view of incisors; underjet. Usually requires incisor table angle adjustment.

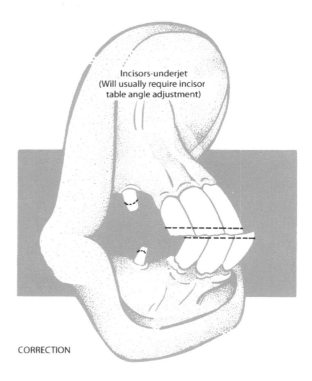

Figure 6-64. Lateral view of incisors; underjet. Usually requires incisor table angle adjustment.

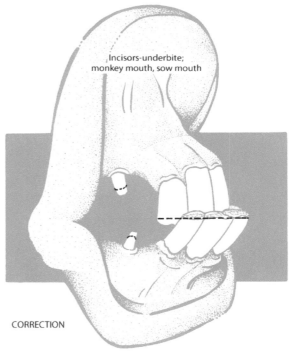

Figure 6-65. Lateral view of incisors; underbite, monkey mouth, sow mouth.

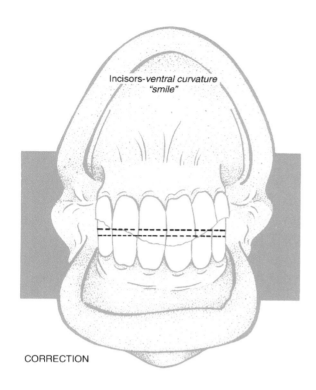

Incisors-*ventral curvature*
"smile"

CORRECTION

Figure 6-66. AP view of incisors; ventral curvature, smile.

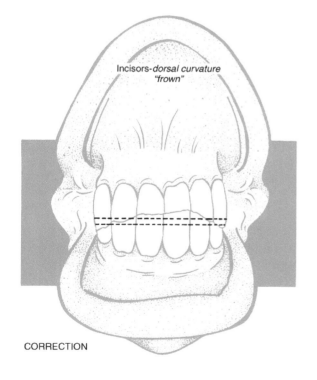

Incisors-*dorsal curvature*
"frown"

CORRECTION

Figure 6-67. AP view of incisors; dorsal curvature, frown.

Regardless of which method and equipment are used, it is essential that the incisors be reduced gradually, taking a little at a time and periodically checking the result. It is important to avoid removing so much length from the incisors that none of the incisors are in occlusion. Creating a gap between the incisor arcades can put excessive pressure on the molars, which may make the horse uncomfortable and cause problems with mastication. Depending on the age of the patient, the amount of reserve crown remaining, and the size of the gap, the deficit created may take a long time to close (by continued incisor eruption). If insufficient reserve crown remains (e.g., in geriatric horses), incisor occlusion may never be restored, which can be disastrous if the molars are expiring or otherwise compromised. To avoid removing too much incisor, I repeat the lateral excursion test during incisor reduction to determine the point at which maximal benefit is obtained.

RECORDKEEPING

On completion of the incisor work, repeat measurements for molar occlusion (lateral excursion test), molar and incisor table angles (if changes were made), and rostro-caudal excursion of the mandible and record the postcorrection findings.

AFTERCARE

Client Instructions

It is relatively uncommon for horses to eat more slowly than normal for a couple of days after extensive dental correction has been performed. It is important to warn the owner or caretaker of this possibility. I infrequently prescribe nonsteroidal antiinflammatory medications for a couple of days in these cases. I may also recommend that the horse be given a few days off work after *extensive* dental correction or following removal of wolf teeth or opening of the gingiva over erupting canine teeth. With the exception of extractions, antibiotics are seldom indicated.

For older horses with expiring or expired teeth, I recommend feeding a complete pelleted ration. If the molars are in such a state that any grinding during mastication is likely to be detrimental, I recommend feeding the pellets as a mash, made by adding water.

Scheduling the Next Appointment

An important part of aftercare that should not be overlooked is scheduling of the next dental examination. The interval may be anywhere from a few weeks to 12 months, depending on the horse's age and particular dental conformation and propensities.

It is common in horses younger than 10 years of age for sharp enamel points to reform and cause buccal ulceration within 4 to 8 months of thorough dental care. So, as a general rule I recommend that young adult horses with no special dental problems receive thorough dental care every 6 months. In horses 3 years of age or younger, buccal ulcerations may reform even sooner than 4 months after dental work. In these patients, I recommend more frequent rechecks (e.g., every 3 to 4 months).

In my experience, sharp enamel points do not recur as quickly in horses older than 10 years as they do in younger horses. Although I recommend semiannual revisits initially in older patients, if there has been little change between visits for at least a year, I recommend extending the interval to 12 months.

*D & B Equine Enterprises, Inc, 207 Silverhill Way NW, Calgary, Alberta, Canada T3B 4K9.

*Carbide Products Co, Torrance, Calif.

*World Wide Equine, Glenns Ferry, Idaho.

*World Wide Equine, Glenns Ferry, Idaho.

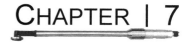

CHAPTER 7

Other Procedures

This chapter discusses dental procedures that can be performed "in the field" but that are not considered routine for most practitioners at this time. The chapter concludes with some specialty procedures that may become routine for some practitioners in the future.

PERORAL EXTRACTION OF PERMANENT CHEEK TEETH

Tom Allen

Permanent cheek teeth that are loose and in need of extraction are a fairly common finding in older horses (midteens and older) (Fig. 7-1). I extract approximately 20 permanent cheek teeth per month in my equine dentistry practice. Although many of these loose teeth can be extracted via the oral cavity in the standing horse, the practitioner should always caution the owner before attempting peroral extraction that in some cases it is impossible to remove all portions of the tooth using this approach. Referral to a surgical facility may become necessary—or may be advisable instead of attempting peroral extraction. *When in doubt* as to your ability to extract a particular tooth in the field, *refer the horse to a surgical facility or to a more experienced practitioner.*

Before proceeding with the extraction, it is also important to discuss with the owner possible complications, postoperative management, and the importance of regular dental maintenance for the remainder of the horse's life. As with any surgical procedure, it is prudent to have the owner sign an informed consent form that outlines these points before proceeding.

Evaluation

The primary indication for extraction of a permanent cheek tooth is excessive looseness, whether caused by a long-standing malocclusion, periodontitis (discussed later), or natural attrition. Unlike infections originating at the tooth root (apical infections), there typically are no outward signs of a problem, such as facial swelling, halitosis, or discharge from the nostrils or skin overlying the affected tooth. Mastication may be affected (e.g., the horse may eat more slowly or drop food while eating), but in most cases the loose tooth is discovered only when the cheek teeth arcades are carefully examined using a full-mouth speculum.

The upper premolars and molars are the most common permanent teeth in need of extraction (Color Plate 55). Expired upper cheek teeth are often encountered in horses older than their midteens. On occasion, these teeth are so loose they can be extracted just with the fingers. More often, however, the tooth is found to be loose only after applying a probe to the occlusal surface and observing the ease with which the tooth can be displaced (either in a buccal-palatal or a rostro-caudal direction) (Fig. 7-2). Gingival separation and periodontal pocket formation are other indications that the tooth is diseased and may be in need of extraction.

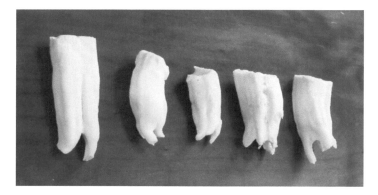

Figure 7-1. Permanent cheek teeth that are loose and in need of extraction are a fairly common finding in older horses (midteens and older).

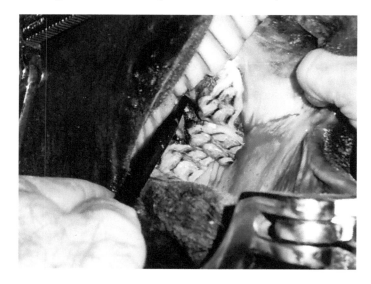

Figure 7-2. Apply a probe to the suspect tooth.

The cheek teeth in the lower arcades require extraction far less often than the uppers. Lower cheek teeth in need of extraction often are obvious by their lingual or buccal displacement. However, some displaced lower cheek teeth are neither loose nor infected, and do not necessarily need to be extracted. It is relatively common for this malalignment to be bilateral. To determine whether a malpositioned cheek tooth is in need of extraction, grasp the tooth with cap extractors or molar extraction forceps and gently twist the tooth back and forth. If the tooth is loose and in need of extraction, just this small amount of movement can be painful during mastication. Compare the movement in the suspected tooth to that which can be demonstrated in adjacent teeth (Fig. 7-3).

Effect of Age

It is important to consider the horse's age when evaluating the mobility of the cheek teeth. In old horses the cheek teeth are somewhat loose compared with those of a younger horse, because the tooth reserve crowns are shorter and narrower, and there is less of a periodontal attachment in old horses (Fig. 7-4). This relative "looseness" is not necessarily an indication of a pathologic condition or of the need for extraction. To determine whether a particular tooth is pathologically loose and in need of extraction, compare it with the same tooth in the other arcade (e.g., compare 109 with 209).

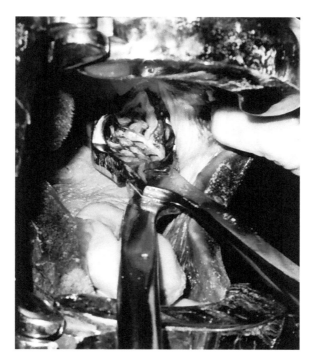

Figure 7-3. Checking the looseness of the 207 with extraction forceps.

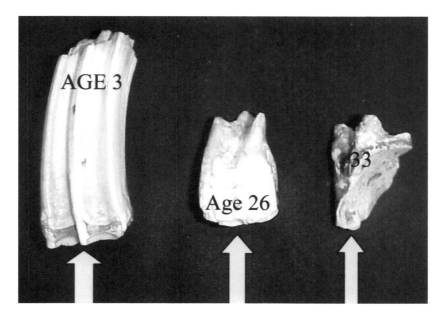

Figure 7-4. Less reserve crown in older teeth. (Courtesy Tony Basile, El Dorado Hills, CA.)

Sedation, Analgesia, and Other Medications

In most instances, the horse is already sedated (having been sedated for dental examination). If not, I sedate the horse using the drugs and dosages outlined in Chapter 3. In addition, I administer morphine sulfate (75 to 150mg IV for a 1000-pound horse), flunixin meglumine (500mg IV for a 1000-pound horse), and, if the horse's tetanus immunization status is in question, tetanus toxoid intramuscularly (IM). Antibiotic coverage may also be a wise precaution.

Extraction Technique

If the tooth is very loose, all that may be required to remove it is to grasp the tooth with molar forceps and remove it from the socket (Fig. 7-5). If the tooth is being held snugly in place by the adjacent teeth and what remains of the periodontal ligament, it may be necessary to use molar spreaders to gradually release the diseased tooth. The molar spreaders are placed as shown in Fig. 7-6 and gradually closed to apply steady pressure on the periodontal ligament of the diseased tooth.

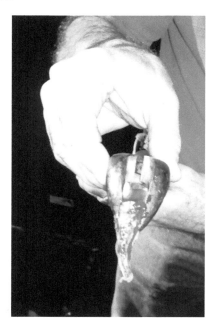

Figure 7-5. If the tooth is very loose, all that may be required to remove it is to grasp the tooth with molar forceps and remove it from the socket.

Once the spreaders can be closed completely between the diseased tooth and its neighbor, the handles are slowly moved from side to side. It works best to exert pressure in one direction and hold for several seconds, then exert pressure on the tooth in the opposite direction and hold, alternating directions until the tooth is sufficiently loose. It may take several minutes of gentle manipulation to loosen the tooth, but patience and persistence are essential. It is easy to break off part of the tooth root by working too quickly or too aggressively.

Once sufficient space has been created using the molar spreaders, molar extraction forceps are used to complete the job. The molar forceps are placed over the crown of the tooth and pressure is applied to the tooth in a buccal-palatal (or buccal-lingual) direction. As with the use of molar spreaders, it is best to move the molar forceps in one direction and hold for several seconds before moving them in the opposite direction. As the tooth loosens, a gentle twisting motion can be added to the side-to-side action (Fig. 7-7).

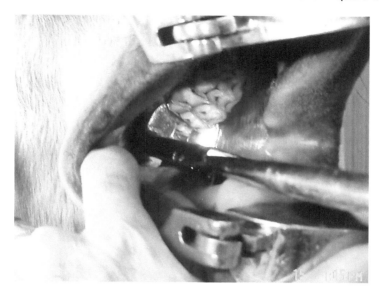

Figure 7-6. Molar spreaders in use.

When the tooth feels sufficiently loose, change the direction of force to a vertical orientation and draw the tooth from the socket. Because the cheek teeth have long roots relative to the crown, in many cases a fulcrum is needed to draw the tooth from the socket. Some molar extraction forceps have a built-in metal fulcrum. Separate fulcrums made of brass can also be purchased.

Inserting a short piece of wooden dowel between the forceps handles and the adjacent tooth makes a simple and effective fulcrum (Color Plate 56). This approach may also be gentler on the teeth, because wood is more "giving" than metal. I keep short sections of dowel of various diameters in my instrument case for this purpose. When needed, I select an appropriately sized piece of dowel and tape it to the molar extractors.

Finishing

Once the tooth is extracted, examine it for completeness and palpate the socket for any root or bone fragments. Then lavage the socket with dilute chlorhexidine solution. To finish, I ease the margins of the teeth rostral and caudal to the empty socket, to remove any sharp edges that may abrade the buccal mucosa or tongue or otherwise cause the horse discomfort.

Common Complications

Probably the most common complication of peroral cheek tooth extraction is fracture of the tooth root. Advising the owner of the possibility of this and other potential complications avoids the ill will that can develop when things don't go according to plan.

Broken Tooth Roots

If part of the tooth root is broken off during manipulation or extraction of the tooth, reasonable attempts should be made to remove the fragment(s). Leaving a portion of tooth root behind may lead to sequestration and abscessation. However, if the root fragment cannot be removed without causing substantial tissue damage, it may be best to leave it in place. Some of these fragments migrate to the gum surface weeks or months later, at which time they can be removed with relative ease if they are causing inflammation. It is important to give the owner the option of referral to a surgical facility for fragment removal.

Abnormally Shaped Tooth Roots

Some teeth that seem very loose are surprisingly difficult to extract. In many of these cases the tooth roots may be abnormally deviated (e.g., curved instead of straight) or there may be an enlargement at the base of the root (Fig. 7-8). By taking the time to loosen the tooth as much as possible and then using a well-placed fulcrum, it is usually possible to extract these abnormal teeth. However, care must be taken to avoid damage to the periodontal bone, the soft tissues, and the adjacent teeth.

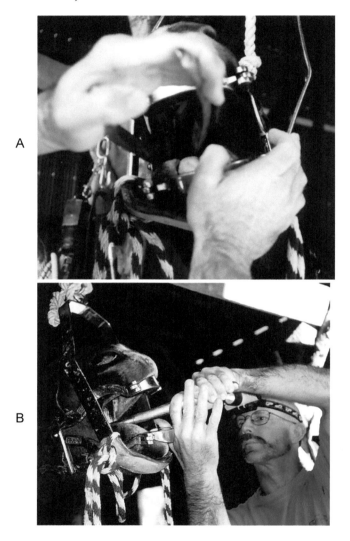

Figure 7-7. A and **B**, As the tooth loosens, gentle twisting motion can be added.

If you feel you cannot remove the tooth without breaking the root or causing damage to adjacent structures, it is best to refer the horse to a surgical facility. If the tooth is very loose, I prescribe antibiotics, antiinflammatory medications (e.g., phenylbutazone), and a complete ration to be fed as a mash until the horse arrives at the surgical facility. Remodeling of bone may occur in 3 to 6 months, allowing completion of extraction *per os* in cases where incomplete extraction is encountered.
Figure 7-7

Aftercare

If some bleeding occurred during the procedure, advise the owner or caretaker that the horse may drop one or two blood clots from the mouth over the next 48 hours. Although it may not be necessary in every case, I routinely prescribe antibiotics (oral trimethoprim-sulfonamide) for 10 to 14 days after extractions.

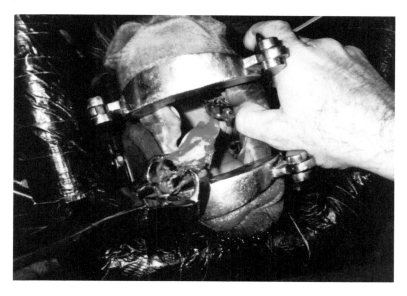

Figure 7-8. Enlargement at the base of root.

I do not pack or plug the tooth socket following peroral extractions of either upper or lower cheek teeth in older horses having short reserve crowns. Plugging the socket minimizes the amount of feed material that can be packed into the socket (contributing to infection and delaying healing). However, plugging the socket seals in any bacteria already in the socket. Also, in many cases the plug material is dislodged too soon to have been of any significant benefit. After extraction, sharp edges of the teeth mesial and distal to the space may need to be addressed (Color Plate 57).

Instead, I simply recommend that the owner feed the horse a complete pelleted ration, made into a mash by adding water, for 3 weeks after extraction. The rationale is that feeding an easily masticated food minimizes the amount of food material that is packed into the socket.

EXTRACTION OF PERMANENT INCISORS

Tom Allen

Loose permanent incisors are encountered far less often than loose permanent cheek teeth. The principles of evaluating the need for extraction are the same for incisors as they are for the cheek teeth (described earlier). It is important to note that in geriatric horses the entire arcade of incisors may be loose, owing to their short, narrow reserve crown. In determining the need for extraction, compare the looseness of the tooth in question with its neighbors or with the corresponding tooth on the opposite side of the mouth.

Loose incisors usually are easily extracted following elevation of the gingival tissue and application of gentle, persistent traction with incisor forceps combined with gentle torsion (Fig. 7-9). This procedure can generally be performed in the standing, sedated horse, as described for peroral extraction of permanent cheek teeth.

NOTE: Never remove an incisor that has been loosened by recent trauma unless it is clear that there is little chance of the tooth remaining viable.

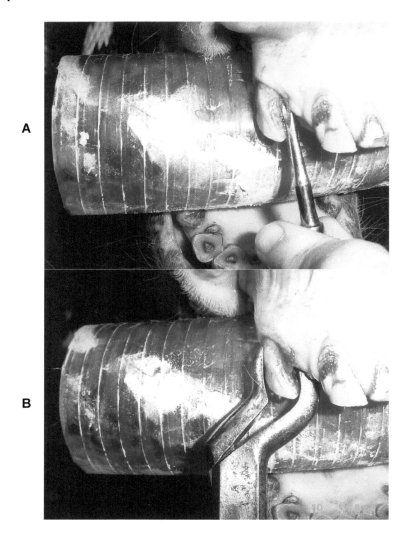

Figure 7-9. A and **B**, Loose incisors are usually easily extracted following elevation of the gingival tissue and application of gentle, persistent traction with incisor forceps.

PERIODONTITIS

Tony Basile

Periodontitis is probably the single greatest cause of premature tooth loss in adult horses. At least 60% of horses older than 15 years of age have some degree of periodontal disease which, if left untreated, could culminate in tooth loss. Although several factors may be involved, one of the primary causes of periodontitis in horses is abnormal masticatory forces on the teeth as a result of malocclusion.

The periodontal ligament and supporting tissues are designed to cope with normal masticatory forces. However, excessive or abnormally directed forces associated with malocclusion can overload the tooth's support system, weakening the periodontal attachment and initiating a destructive cascade of inflammation and degeneration.

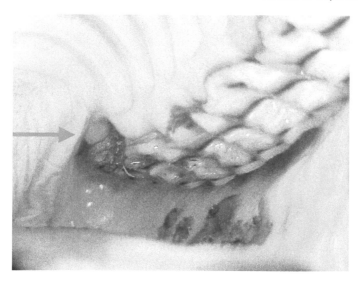

Figure 7-10. Impaction of food in periodontal pocket. (*Courtesy Tony Basile, El Dorado Hills, CA.*)

Stages of Disease

Untreated, periodontitis is a continuum of periodontal inflammation and degeneration. Initially the response to abnormal occlusal forces may be restricted (at least clinically) to gingivitis and the formation of a small gap (a diastema) between the normally tightly packed cheek teeth. (Diastemata also form between the cheek teeth in geriatric horses because the reserve crown narrows as the tooth nears the end of its functional life.)

Impaction of food material into the widened gingival sulcus and into the spaces between the teeth (the interproximate spaces) exacerbates the problem and leads to formation of periodontal pockets beside and between the teeth. Pressure from the impacted feed material and the action of bacterial toxins damage the periodontal attachments further, eventually resulting in lysis of the alveolar bone and excessive loosening of the tooth (Fig. 7-10).

The stages of periodontal disease are listed in Box 7-1. It is important to note that different areas of the mouth can be affected by different stages of the disease (Figs. 7-11 and 7-12).

Diagnosis

Clinically significant periodontal disease is identified predominantly in horses older than 15 years of age; however, the propensity may be established at a much earlier age. External signs of periodontitis variably include abnormal mastication, halitosis, hypersalivation, and loss of body condition. However, horses with clinically significant periodontal disease may show no obvious signs. Thus diagnosis of periodontitis requires careful examination of the oral cavity using a full-mouth speculum, a good light source, and some type of dental probe.

Gingivitis

Inflammation of the gingiva is commonly found in horses. The gingiva is reddened and bleeds readily with only slight provocation (e.g., during routine floating). Gingivitis may be localized to a single tooth or series of teeth, or it may involve the entire arcade or even the whole mouth.

Box 7-1	Stages of Periodontal Disease
Stage 1	Gingival inflammation is the primary lesion. There may be some degree of gingi - val recession from the base of the tooth, and calculus accumulation. Narrow interproximate spaces containing some food particles may be found at the base of the teeth; however, the food material does not prevent contact of adjacent molars.
Stage 2	Impaction of food material in the widening interproximate space prevents contact between adjacent molars for part of their length. When the diastema is irrigated and débrided, there are no visible periodontal pockets, although there is a slight amount of gingival recession.
Stage 3	Adjacent molars are slightly separated along their entire length by impaction of feed material in the widened interproximate space. When the diastema is irrigated and débrided, shallow periodontal pockets (1 to 2mm deep) are found at the base of the teeth; débridement causes some bleeding.
Stage 4	Adjacent molars are clearly separated by feed impaction in the now substantial interproximate space. The tooth may be slightly loose. When the diastema is irrigated and débrided, deep periodontal pockets (>2mm deep) are found.
Stage 5	Food is packed around the base of the tooth, which is loose and may be displaced.

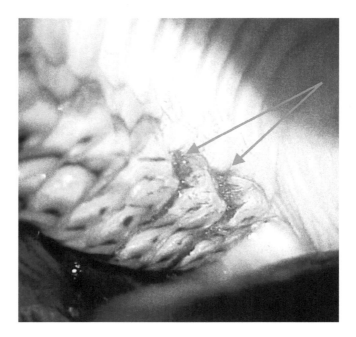

Figure 7-11. Another example of a periodontal pocket. (*Courtesy Tony Basile, El Dorado Hills, CA.*)

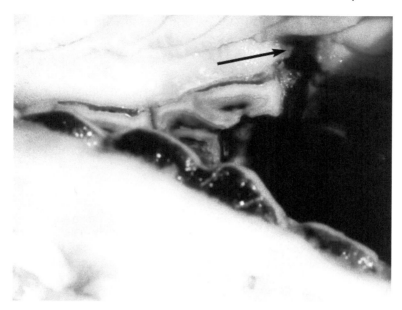

Figure 7-12. Example of stage 4. (*Courtesy Tony Basile, El Dorado Hills, CA.*)

Periodontal Pockets

Periodontal pockets are most obvious along the buccal and lingual-palatal sides of the tooth, although they are as common in the interproximate spaces. Periodontitis in the interproximate area is potentially more destructive, because early signs of periodontitis in this sheered location can be difficult to detect. Destruction of the periodontal attachments may be advanced by the time periodontitis is identified in the interproximate space. Failure to recognize and address these periodontal pockets is a common reason why otherwise appropriate treatment for periodontitis fails to protect the tooth from loosening and loss.

Gingivitis, accumulation of food material, and periodontal pocket formation on the buccal and lingual-palatal sides of the tooth are easily identified using a full-mouth speculum, a good light source, and a blunt dental probe. An intraoral mirror can be useful for examining the periodontal areas in the caudal parts of the mouth.

Interproximate periodontitis should be suspected in any horse with malocclusion involving the cheek teeth arcades. It is suggested in specific locations by finding food material between adjacent teeth, excessive mobility of a particular tooth, or discharge from the interproximate space following burring or floating of the occlusal surfaces using motorized instruments.

Calculus

Calculus (tartar) is the tannish-brown conglomeration of organic and inorganic material that can accumulate on the surface of the teeth, most often the incisors, canines, and buccal aspects of the cheek teeth. Calculus accumulation alone rarely leads to severe periodontal disease or tooth loss. However, calculus adjacent to the gingival margin causes or contributes to gingivitis.

Instruments for Treating Periodontitis

Hand Picks and Scalers

Hand picks and scalers are useful for removing calculus and for removing feed material and other debris from the interproximate space. However, many of these instruments are too wide to fit into the narrow interproximate space in horses with mild or early periodontitis (Color Plate 58).

Ultrasonic Scalers

Ultrasonic scalers are excellent for removing large accumulations of calculus. Most units include a lavage feature to irrigate the area during scaling. Care must be taken to avoid overheating or otherwise damaging the tooth and periodontal tissues with these instruments. With currently available units, the handpieces are too short to reach the back of the horse's mouth, and the tips do not allow access to the interproximate space in many horses. Another drawback is that replacement tips are expensive.

Pressurized Lavage and Débridement

The Equine Dental System* is specifically designed for treating periodontal disease in horses. Its long hand piece allows access to the caudalmost cheek teeth. The unit can be used with dilute chlorhexidine solution for lavage; with sodium bicarbonate solution as a mild abrasive for calculus removal; or with 25-micron aluminum oxide for more abrasive cleaning. (When using aluminum oxide, care must be taken to avoid damaging the periodontal cementum.) Pressure output can be varied, so even deep periodontal pockets can be safely and effectively lavaged. A suction function allows removal of debris from deep pockets as they are being lavaged (Fig. 7-13).

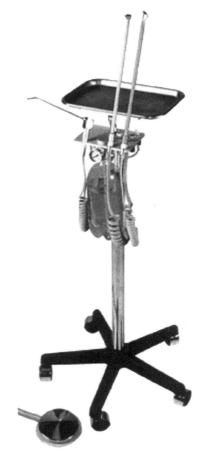

Figure 7-13. Air abrasion unit. (*Courtesy Tony Basile, El Dorado Hills, CA.*)

Treatment of Periodontitis

The goals of treatment are to arrest the process, preserve the remaining periodontal attachments, and thus save the tooth from premature loss. The effectiveness of periodontal therapy is made possible by the remarkable regenerative capacity of the periodontal tissues when the underlying problem is addressed. Although the specifics of treatment vary with the stage of the disease, the principles of periodontal therapy are the same:

1. Address crown height and table angle in all arcades to normalize occlusion as much as possible.
2. Remove all feed material and other debris from the interproximate spaces and periodontal pockets.

Some horses require additional therapy, repeated débridement, and regular dental equilibration to correct periodontitis or manage its recurrence.

Stages 1 and 2

Optimizing occlusion may be all that is required to resolve periodontitis that is limited to gingival inflammation. Irrigation with water or 0.1% chlorhexidine solution is indicated for any areas in which food material has accumulated at the base of the teeth. A syringe with a 16-gauge needle attached makes a useful water pic for this procedure. A dental pick or similar instrument may be needed to remove feed material that is packed into the interproximate space; the space should then be vigorously lavaged. Any calculus should be removed as described later.

Stages 3 to 5

The interproximate spaces and periodontal pockets should be thoroughly irrigated and débrided to remove all feed material and necrotic tissue. (Slight bleeding from the inflamed gingiva can be expected following lavage or débridement.) An oral antibiotic gel* can then be applied to the periodontal pockets (Color Plate 59). If the periodontitis is not too advanced, it may resolve just with this treatment and dental equilibration. Provided the malocclusion can be corrected, the diastema should narrow or disappear.

With deep periodontal pockets and extensive diastemata, it is often a good idea to pack the pockets and entire interproximate space with dental impression material† to prevent further impaction with feed material. Horses with deep periodontal pockets should be reevaluated and treated every 10 to 14 days until resolution is well underway. Frequent reevaluation (e.g., every 1 to 3 months) is then indicated. In horses with severe periodontal disease, extraction of the loose tooth may be the best option.

Calculus Removal

Calculus can be removed using a hand scaler, an ultrasonic scaler, or air abrasion (Fig. 7-14). Care must be taken to avoid traumatizing the gingiva. Although calculus removal is a useful adjunct to specific periodontal therapy, it may be insufficient alone for the treatment of periodontitis. Also, new calculus formation is evident in as little as 10 days after scaling in some horses.

In horses with a particular propensity for forming calculus, instructing the client to brush the horse's accessible teeth (incisors, canines, and rostral cheek teeth) each day may prevent calculus formation and associated gingivitis. Most horses can be trained to stand and tolerate having their teeth brushed with a soft-bristle toothbrush and sodium bicarbonate.

Prevention of Periodontitis

The incidence of periodontal disease and consequent tooth loss can be minimized by preventing or promptly correcting malocclusions. Thorough examination of the horse's dental arcades should begin when the permanent teeth are beginning to erupt and should continue regularly throughout the horse's life. Maleruptions, malalignments, and malformations should be addressed as they develop.

DENTAL RESTORATION TECHNIQUES

Tony Basile

Restoration of diseased permanent teeth is a relatively new concept in equine dentistry. Procedures aimed at preserving diseased teeth are being adapted from human and small animal dentistry for use in horses. As procedures and instruments are developed further, restoration techniques may become more commonplace and thus substantially decrease the need for extractions.

Incisor Restoration

Incisor restoration techniques are being developed to preserve fractured, carious, or otherwise abnormal permanent incisors. Indications include protection of an exposed pulp cavity, fracture repair, and restoration or improvement of occlusion (Fig. 7-15).

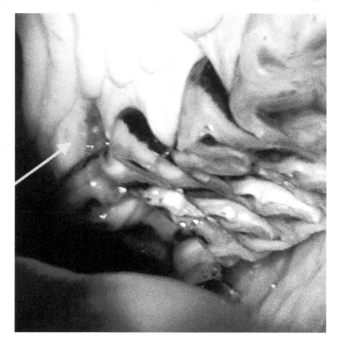

Figure 7-14. Stage 4 of periodontal disease. (*Courtesy Tony Basile, El Dorado Hills, CA.*)

Infundibular Filling of the Cheek Teeth

Filling of deep infundibula in the cheek teeth can delay or prevent cupping, fracture, and decay of these teeth. The need for infundibular filling is determined by examining the occlusal surfaces of the cheek teeth for the following abnormalities:
- Blackening of the enamel; in advanced stages the enamel may be missing in some areas
- Pitting of the infundibulum, with accumulation of food particles in the crater (Fig. 7-16)
- Foul odor (especially from the debris in the infundibulum)

In advanced stages the center of the tooth is eroded and the infundibula coalesce into one large crater (Fig. 7-17).

Infundibular filling is most appropriate for teeth with moderate to severe decay, in horses younger than 20 years of age. In older horses, the tooth may be too close to expiring for this procedure to be worthwhile.

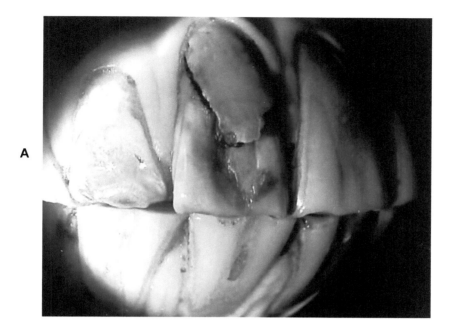

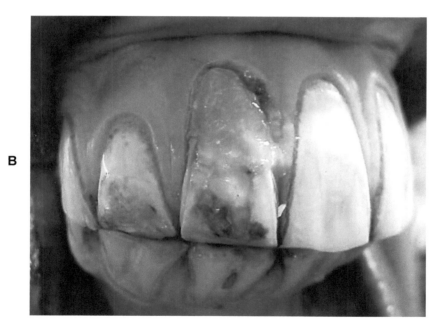

Figure 7-15. A, Before restoration. **B**, After restoration. (*Courtesy Tony Basile, El Dorado Hills, CA.*)

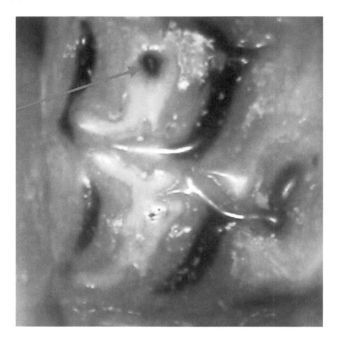

Figure 7-16. Pitting of infundibulum. (*Courtesy Tony Basile, El Dorado Hills, CA.*)

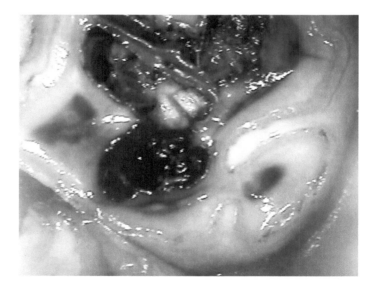

Figure 7-17. Necrotic infundibulum. (*Courtesy Tony Basile, El Dorado Hills, CA.*)

The technique is similar to that used by human and small animal dentists. The infundibulum is thoroughly cleaned of any impacted feed material using a dental PIC and compressed air. The infundibular walls are then carefully débrided with a dental drill. Acid etching of the infundibular walls ensures good bonding and retention of the composite resin, which is used to fill the entire cavity of the infundibulum. Finally, the surface of the composite is contoured and a layer of sealant is applied (Color Plate 60).

CORRECTION OF BRACHYGNATHISM IN FOALS

Michael Boero

Brachygnathism (overbite; "parrot mouth") is a malocclusion in which the mandible is shorter than the maxilla. The malocclusion may involve only the incisors or both the incisors and the cheek teeth. The condition may be present at birth or develop as the foal grows. Routine examination of the dental arcades in young foals is important for early detection of this and other oral abnormalities.

Correction Techniques

Methods of correction for brachygnathism in foals vary with the severity of the malocclusion. Regardless of whether orthodontic devices are used, frequent dental maintenance is important. Specifically, any problems involving the cheek teeth that may inhibit rostral movement of the mandible should be diligently corrected. Also, unopposed and overgrown portions of the incisors should be reduced as needed to prevent "locking" of the lower incisors behind the uppers.

Wiring

If the upper and lower incisors are in partial contact, the upper incisors may be wired to the upper premolars to retard growth of the maxilla until the mandible "catches up." This procedure is performed under general anesthesia; but because it is not a sterile surgery, it can be done in the field.

Acrylic Orthodontic Devices

In foals in which the upper incisors completely overshoot the lowers (i.e., no contact between upper and lower incisors), some type of orthodontic device is needed in addition to wiring. The orthodontic device is used to prevent ventral drifting of the premaxilla and to keep the lower incisors from becoming locked behind the upper incisors (Color Plate 61).

There are three types of orthodontic device used for correction of brachygnathism in foals:

1. A removable acrylic plate that the foal wears like a bit. The device is removed when the foal eats, so owner compliance is needed.
2. A fixed acrylic device, custom-made and fitted after taking a plaster model of the foal's incisors. This method provides good documentation of the condition before treatment. However, the foal must be anesthetized twice and the procedure is technically difficult.
3. A fixed acrylic device, molded in place at the same time the upper incisors are wired. With this device the acrylic is placed behind the upper incisors to prevent the lower incisors from becoming locked behind the uppers. The wires help hold the orthodontic device in place. The acrylic is molded so that it is slightly thicker caudally, creating a plane that slopes downward from caudal to rostral. The lower incisors are thus encouraged to move rostrally when they are in contact with the acrylic plate. The device may need to be replaced periodically as the foal grows, and if a wire or the acrylic plate breaks.

Regardless of which method is used, it is important to start treatment early, while there is sufficient growth potential for mandibular bone growth to correct the disparity. For this reason, examination of foals' mouths should be routine, starting early in the foal's life and continuing regularly throughout the growth period. It is also important to address the entire mouth when treating this incisor abnormality.

*Pacific Equine Dental Institute Inc, 7118 Cinnamon Teal Way, El Dorado Hills, CA 95762.

*Doxyrobe Gel, Pharmacia & Upjohn, 7000 Portage Road, Kalamazoo, MI 49001.

†Sullivan-Schein Dental, 135 Duryea Road, Melville, NY 11747.

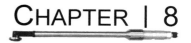

CHAPTER 8

Dentistry in Miniature Horses

Carl Mitz and Tom Allen

Miniature horses (minis) have become very popular in recent years. Because most of these tiny horses are companion animals rather than performance animals, their dental needs are often overlooked. However, minis experience the same types of dental abnormalities described for larger horses. In fact, owing to the practice of breeding for small size ("the smaller the better") and extensive inbreeding, maleruptions, malformations, and malocclusions are much more common and tend to be much more severe in minis than in larger breeds. These problems are particularly common in minis less than 28 inches in height (Color Plate 62).

As a general rule, minis require more frequent dental care and more extensive dental corrections, starting at a much younger age, than do most larger horses. Because the mini's teeth are approximately the same size as those of a 1000-pound horse (Fig. 8-1), overcrowding in both the incisor and molar arcades is a very common problem in minis. The maleruptions and malocclusions that result require earlier and more aggressive intervention than most of the less dramatic malocclusions in larger breeds. Thus several dental procedures are routinely performed in minis that are seldom, if ever, required in larger horses.

(NOTE: Although this chapter focuses on miniature horses, the same principles apply to miniature donkeys and miniature mules.)

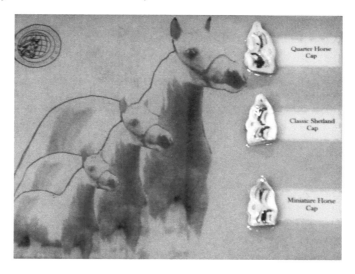

Figure 8-1. Minis' teeth are approximately the same size as those of a 1000-pound horse. (*Courtesy Tami Mitz, Brenham, TX.*)

CHALLENGES OF MINIATURE HORSE DENTISTRY

Miniature horses present some unique challenges to the dental practitioner:
- Small stature—minis can be difficult to restrain effectively and difficult to work on comfortably and efficiently without straining the practitioner's knees and/or back.
- Temperament—minis can be volatile, even explosive; they are not always well trained (many novice owners succumb to the "cuteness" factor in disciplining willful minis).
- Shape and size of the head—the short mandibles and maxillae predispose to several dental abnormalities that, once established, can be very difficult to improve; there is very little room to work in these small, overcrowded mouths.
- Dental development—dental eruption times are delayed and highly variable, compared with larger breeds; full-size teeth in a "miniaturized" skull make maleruptions and malocclusions common.
- Sedation—sedation is often needed for procedures other than routine floating; the dosage required is highly variable (from a fraction of the per-pound dosage routinely used in larger horses to twice that dosage).
- Dental instruments—few dental instruments are designed for these small patients.

Despite these challenges and practical difficulties, miniature horse dentistry affords the practitioner a wealth of opportunities for studying dental pathology. It can also be very rewarding, because appropriately timed interventions during the young horse's formative years can have life-long benefits.

EQUIPMENT

Performing proper dentistry in minis is akin to building a ship in a bottle: access is always a challenge; and skill and patience are needed in equal parts. Currently, few manufacturers are making equine dental equipment specifically for small patients, although this situation is changing. Small full-mouth specula for minis and small ponies are already available or can be custom-made. Some full-size specula can be used on minis, too. The incisor plates are much wider than needed, but provided the speculum allows adjustment of the jaw angle in very small increments, full-size specula can be comfortably used in small patients.

The low-profile, slimline hand floats and many of the motorized burrs and floats designed for use in larger horses can be used in minis. Pneumatic dental instruments are particularly useful. Reciprocating pneumatic floats come in a wide selection of shaft angles and lengths, and they make shaping the molar arcades much easier on both the patient and the practitioner. Because this float is quiet and has a smooth action, routine dental procedures can be performed without sedation in most minis. Small, high-speed pneumatic burrs also make short work of molar reductions in these small mouths (Figs. 8-2 to 8-5).

Unless the patient can be restrained on a raised work area, a good set of knee pads is a worthwhile investment. Dental work can be performed while the practitioner is seated on a stool; however, the patient must be well restrained. In Dr. Allen's practice, work on small patients has been made much easier by customizing a horse trailer into a mobile equine dental clinic (see Chapter 2). For small patients, a platform is slipped into the stocks and the patient is walked onto the platform and restrained with two straps (one over the back and one behind the rump) (see Color Plate 62).

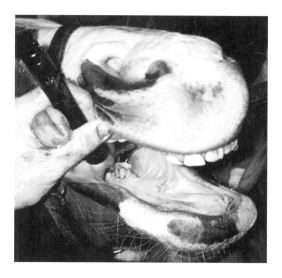

Color Plate 51. Obvious #706 cap (on #306 premolar).

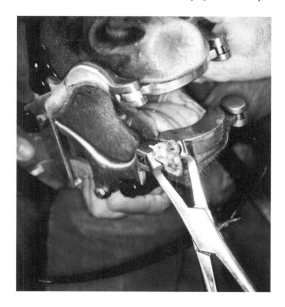

Color Plate 52. Number 6 cap removed.

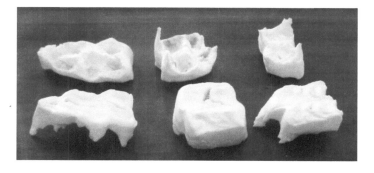

Color Plate 53. Assorted premolar caps.

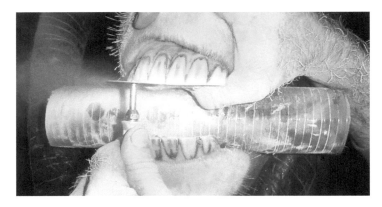

Color Plate 54. Dust produced by incisor work.

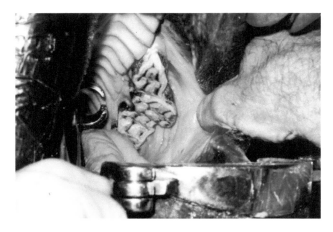

Color Plate 55. The upper premolars and molars are the most common permanent teeth in need of extraction. This tooth (number 207) is obviously loose and in need of extraction.

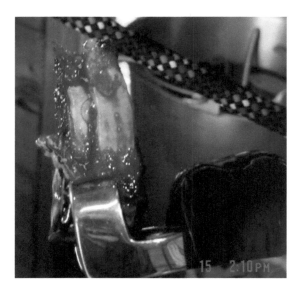

Color Plate 56. Inserting a short piece of wooden dowel between the forceps handles and the adjacent tooth makes a simple and effective fulcrum.

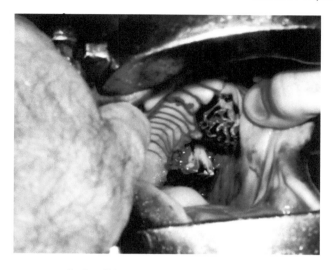

Color Plate 57. After extraction.

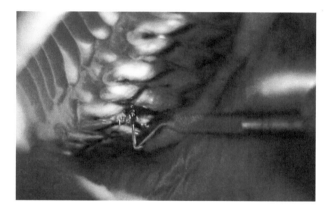

Color plate 58. Using an explorer to measure the depth of the cavity (color-coded in 3-mm increments). *(Courtesy Tony Basile, El Dorado Hills, CA.)*

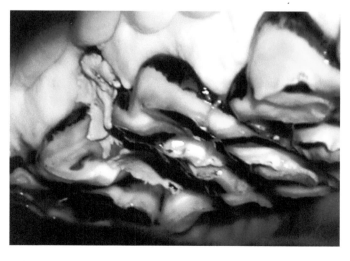

Color Plate 59. Gel in place. *(Courtesy Tony Basile, El Dorado Hills, CA.)*

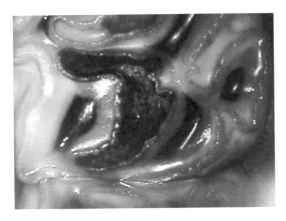 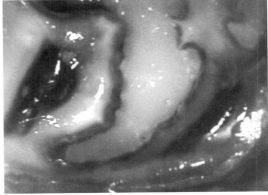

Color Plate 60. A, Before filling. **B,** After filling (Courtesy Tony Basile, El Dorado Hills, CA.)

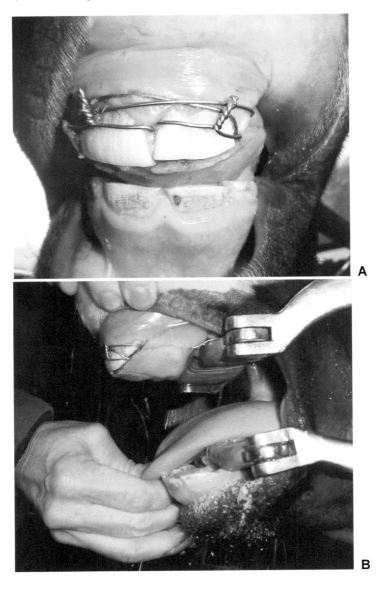

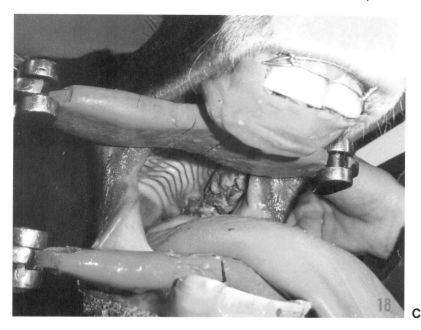

C

Color Plate 61 cont'd. A-C, The orthodontic device is used to prevent ventral drifting of the premaxilla and to keep the lower incisors from becoming locked behind the upper incisors.

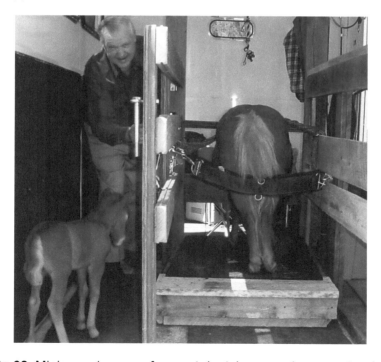

Color Plate 62. Minis require more frequent dental care and more extensive dental corrections because of their small body size and large teeth.

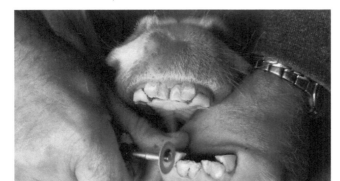

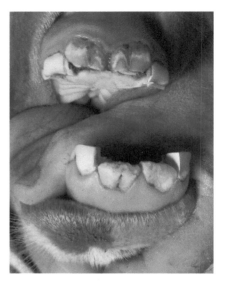

Color Plate 63. A, (Before) in minis approaching 3 years of age, space for the erupting permanent 1s can be made by trimming the mesial portions of the deciduous 2s. **B**, After treatment. (*Courtesy of Tami Mitz, Brenhan, TX.*)

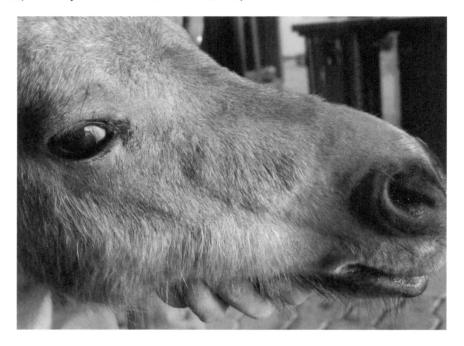

Color Plate 64. Owing to the small size and refined shape of the head, mandibular or maxillary swellings associated with eruption of the permanent cheek teeth (eruption cysts) are very common in young minis. (*Courtesy Tami Mitz, Brenham, TX.*)

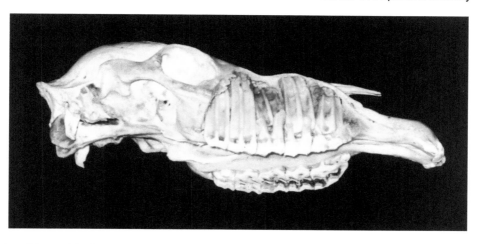

Color Plate 65. Skull showing the effects of eruption cysts. (*Courtesy Tami Mitz, Brenham, TX.*)

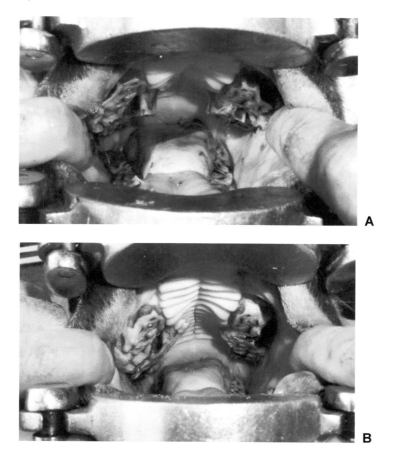

Color Plate 66. A, Displaced palatally are 108 and 208, before dentistry. **B**, After the 108 has been reduced and the 207 extracted. (*Courtesy Tami Mitz, Brenham, TX.*)

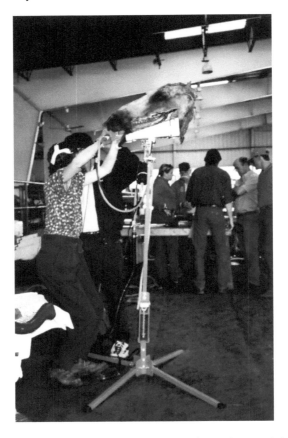

Color Plate 67. Dr. Kristen Wilewski demonstrating at a wet lab for the IAED annual meeting, 2002.

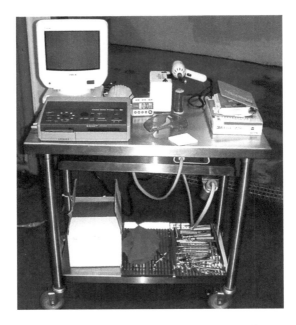

Color Plate 68. Equipment for advanced dentistry techniques. (*Courtesy Tony Basile, El Dorado Hills, CA.*)

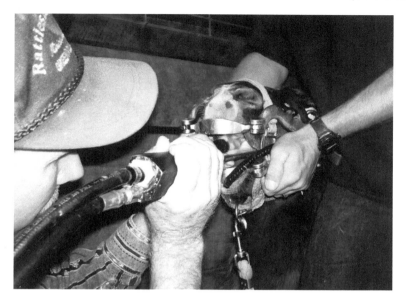

Figure 8-2. Pneumatic dental instruments are particularly useful.

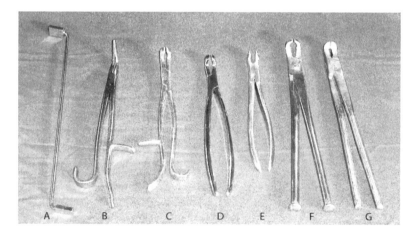

Figure 8-3. Cap and molar extractors (left to right): **A**, Fulcrum. **B**, Molar fragment forceps. **C**, Reynolds cap forceps. **D**, Closed-head forceps. **E**, Open-head forceps. **F**, Closed-head molar forceps. **G**, Small-headed molar spreaders. (*Courtesy Tami Mitz, Brenham, TX.*)

INCISORS

In larger breeds, the median times for eruption of the deciduous incisors are as follows: 1 week for the 1s (centrals), 5 weeks for the 2s (laterals), and 8 months for the 3s (corners). However, in minis, average eruption times are 1 month, 4 months, and 12 months for the 1s, 2s, and 3s, respectively.

In addition to the overall delay in eruption times, opposing incisors often erupt at different times (Fig. 8-6). When a disparity is found in the eruption of an opposing pair of deciduous incisors, eruption of the retarded incisor can be encouraged by incising the gingiva over the unerupted tooth. At the same time, the crown of the erupted opposing tooth can be slightly reduced in height so that it does not impede or overwhelm the erupting tooth.

Eruption of the permanent incisors in minis is also delayed compared with larger breeds and is quite variable. In general, the smaller the horse, the later the deciduous teeth are shed and the permanent teeth erupt. In many minis the deciduous incisors are shed by the erupting permanent incisors at 3, 4, and 5 years of age for the 1s, 2s, and 3s, respectively.

Maleruptions, malformations, and malocclusions involving the incisors are very common in minis. Because these problems begin at an early age, it is extremely important to *begin regular dental exams in the first few months of a foal's life* if these problems are to be prevented or corrected.

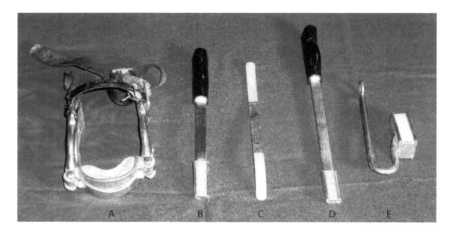

Figure 8-4. A, Mini speculum. **B,** Upturned gritted float blade. **C,** S-file. **D,** Straight gritted blade float. **E,** Wedge. (*Courtesy Tami Mitz, Brenham, TX.*)

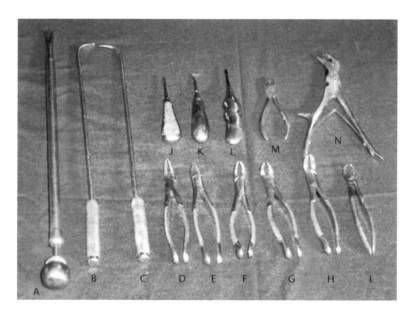

Figure 8-5. Extracting instruments. **A,** Blind loss chisel. **B,** Spade dental pick. **C,** Pointed dental pick. **D,** Angle forceps. **E,** Fragments forceps. **F,** Angled premolar forceps. **G,** Straight premolar forceps. **H,** Splitting forceps. **I,** Cow horn forceps. **J,** Serrated elevator. **K,** Angle elevator. **L,** Straight elevator. **M,** Small cutter. **N,** Double action rongeur. (*Courtesy Tami Mitz, Brenham, TX.*)

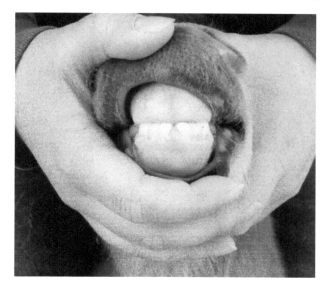

Figure 8-6. Foal without top teeth. (*Courtesy Tami Mitz, Brenham, TX.*)

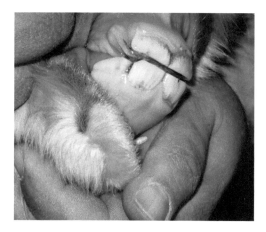

Figure 8-7. There is simply not enough room for all of the incisors to erupt in their proper location in many cases. (*Courtesy Tami Mitz, Brenham, TX.*)

Overcrowded Incisor Arcades

Because the head is so narrow, overcrowding of the incisor arcades is very common in minis. There is simply not enough room for all of the incisors to erupt in their proper location in many cases (Fig. 8-7). Depending on the age of the patient, space can be created and overcrowding avoided by extracting or trimming some of the deciduous incisors.

Extraction of Deciduous Teeth

If a deciduous incisor is extracted before the horse is 16 months old, it will not be replaced by a permanent tooth. Removal of the deciduous tooth at an early age evidently causes sufficient damage to the bud of the underlying permanent tooth that the tooth fails to develop. This fact can be used to advantage to prevent overcrowding of the incisor arcades. Some minis are better off with four pairs of incisors, instead of six (Fig. 8-8). Early extraction of all four deciduous 3s can achieve this goal simply and relatively atraumatically.

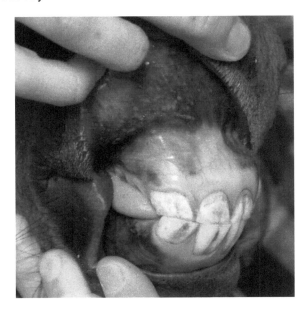

Figure 8-8. Some minis are better off with four pairs of incisors instead of six. (*Courtesy Tami Mitz, Brenham, TX.*)

Deciduous incisors are fairly easy to extract using a small dental elevator and splitting forceps. The gingiva is separated from the tooth using the elevator. Splitting forceps are then used to create a gap between the tooth and its neighbor. Once the tooth is sufficiently loose, it is extracted with the forceps, using the adjacent tooth as a fulcrum. The crown of the deciduous incisor is much larger than the apex, so once the tooth is loosened in this way it is easily extracted.

Trimming To Create Space

In minis approaching 3 years of age, space for the erupting permanent 1s can be made by trimming the mesial portions of the deciduous 2s (Color Plate 63). The need for this procedure is evident when a deciduous 1 is shed and it is apparent that the mesial portion of the deciduous 2 will impede the erupting permanent 1. The easiest way to trim these teeth is with the edge of a diamond cut-off wheel. Care must be taken not to damage the gum or any soft tissue caudal to the tooth (e.g., the palatal mucosa or tongue).

Typically, horses that don't have enough space for the 1s also won't have enough space for the 2s or 3s. But rather than trimming the deciduous 3s when the permanent 2s are due to erupt (at around 4 years of age), it is generally best simply to remove the deciduous 3s, as described earlier. If the foal is older than 16 months of age, the permanent 3s will still erupt; in fact, they will erupt earlier than normal. However, there should be plenty of room for the permanent 2s in the meantime. If space is an issue for the erupting permanent 3s, they can be managed as described later (Fig. 8-9).

Malpositioned or Malformed 3s

Eruption of the permanent 3s usually does not take place until the mini is 5 years old. If overcrowding was not addressed earlier, many of these permanent 3s are malpositioned or malformed. There are two options for managing abnormal 3s: reshape them to a more normal tooth shape, or extract them. There will be cases in which the tooth is so malpositioned that extraction is the best option for the horse (Figs. 8-10 and 8-11).

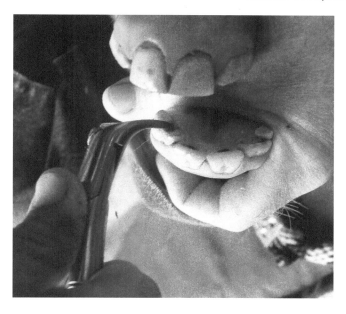

Figure 8-9. It is generally best simply to remove the deciduous 3s. (*Courtesy Tami Mitz, Brenham, TX.*)

Extraction of Permanent Incisors

Extraction of permanent incisors in minis is as described in Chapter 7. A dental elevator is used to free the gingival attachments and as much of the periodontal ligament from the tooth as possible. Extraction forceps are then used to steadily apply tension and torque to the tooth until it is loose enough to be drawn from the socket.

Supernumerary Incisors

It is common in minis for one or more deciduous incisors to be retained, causing the permanent incisor to erupt caudal to the deciduous tooth. This problem can involve only one tooth, several teeth, or an entire incisor arcade, resulting in a double row of incisors (Fig. 8-12).

When just one or a few teeth are involved, the best approach is to extract the deciduous incisor(s), as described earlier. Doing so allows the permanent incisor(s) to migrate labially into a more normal position.

In horses with a complete double set of incisors in one or both arcades, it is generally best to leave the retained deciduous incisors in place. Then just shorten and shape the entire incisor arcade (both deciduous and permanent incisors) as needed to optimize prehension and both lateral and rostro-caudal excursion of the mandible. If the entire row of retained deciduous incisors is extracted, there is a chance that not all of the permanent incisors will migrate into their normal position. The resulting malocclusion may be more problematic than the double row of incisors.

Unopposed Incisors

There are four situations in which the incisors may be unopposed in minis:
- Monkey or sow mouth (underbite, undershot jaw)
- Parrot mouth (overbite, overshot jaw)
- Missing incisors
- Malpositioned incisors

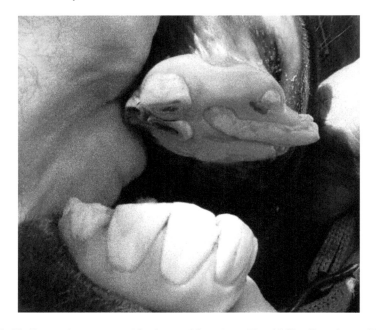

Figure 8-10. Malformed permanent incisors. (*Courtesy Tami Mitz, Brenham, TX.*)

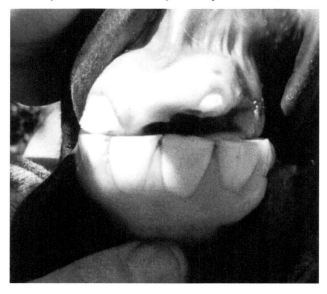

Figure 8-11. Extracted malformed incisors. (*Courtesy Tami Mitz, Brenham, TX.*)

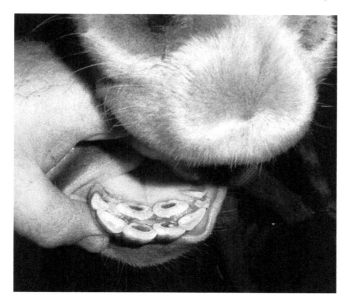

Figure 8-12. Double row of incisors. (*Courtesy Tami Mitz, Brenham, TX.*)

Monkey Mouth in Adults

Monkey mouth is very common in minis (Figs. 8-13 and 8-14). In adults, the defect is managed by shortening the lower incisors to just above the gingiva, being careful not to expose the pulp chamber. The upper incisors are shortened only as necessary to prevent them from contacting the mandible and to optimize lateral excursion of the molar arcades. (The upper incisors have a tendency to become V-shaped and lock into the mandible.)

The molar arcades should also be examined, with special attention paid to the lower 6s. In almost all minis with monkey mouth, the lower 6s have ramps (see Chapter 5) or the entire tooth is overgrown, depending on the degree of disparity between the mandible and the maxilla. The lower 6s should be reduced in height as needed to level the occlusal surface, and the rostral border should be rounded as described for bit seats in Chapter 6.

In addition to lower 6 ramps or overgrowth, the upper 11s may be overlong or have caudal hooks that can ulcerate the cheek, gum, or tongue. Correction of upper 11 hooks is as described in Chapter 6. Horses with monkey mouth require frequent, thorough dental care.

Monkey Mouth in Foals

In many cases this abnormality can be prevented or corrected by examining the foal in the first 3 to 4 months of life and making appropriate dental corrections. The goal is to remove any hindrances to rostro-caudal movement of the mandible relative to the maxilla. The cheek teeth (deciduous 6, 7, and 8) are floated to remove any hooks, points, or ridges that might "lock" the molar arcades, limiting rostro-caudal movement. In addition, the rostral portion of the deciduous 6s should be shortened and rounded (as described for bit seats in Chapter 6) to decrease the potential for rostral hook formation in the coming months.

Correction is best achieved using a full-mouth speculum and either small hand floats or a small motorized burr. Care must be taken not to excessively smooth the occlusal surface nor remove too much tooth; the deciduous premolars are relatively soft and crown is easily removed. Finally, the incisors should be shortened so that there is a gap of approximately 1mm between the upper and lower incisor arcades. Temporarily taking the incisors out of occlusion prevents "locking" of the incisor arcades that might impede jaw growth and dental development.

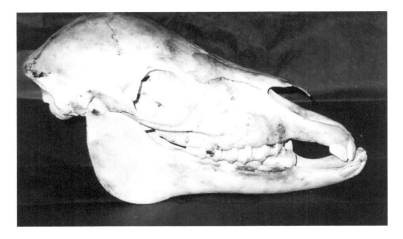

Figure 8-13. Monkey mouth skull. (*Courtesy Tami Mitz, Brenham, TX.*)

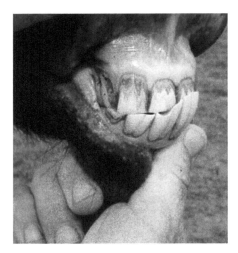

Figure 8-14. Monkey mouth. (*Courtesy Tami Mitz, Brenham, TX.*)

These procedures are most successful in preventing or correcting bite abnormalities if the foal is allowed to graze following correction. Regardless, young horses must be rechecked frequently during the first 3 years of life and dental corrections made as needed to keep all arcades resistance-free. Some foals will need dental correction repeatedly, whereas others may require only the initial treatment. Most cases are corrected with conscientious dental maintenance. However, in a small percentage of foals the defect cannot be corrected with any amount of dental equilibration. These are the cases that may benefit from application of retention wires, similar to the procedures described for correction of brachygnathism in Chapter 7.

Parrot Mouth

Parrot mouth is rare in minis (Fig. 8-15). When this malocclusion is found, it can be managed by shortening the upper incisors until the tables extend slightly below the palate mucosa, being careful not to expose the pulp chamber. The lower incisors are shortened only as necessary to prevent them from contacting the palate mucosa. Prevention of parrot mouth is based on the same principles described earlier for the prevention of monkey mouth: eliminate any hindrances to rostro-caudal movement of the mandible relative to the maxilla.

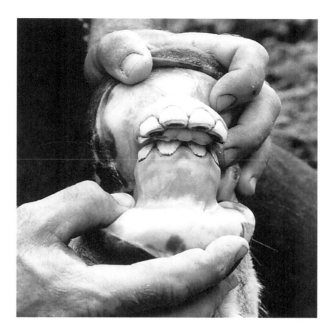

Figure 8-15. Parrot mouth is rare in minis. (*Courtesy Tami Mitz, Brenham, TX.*)

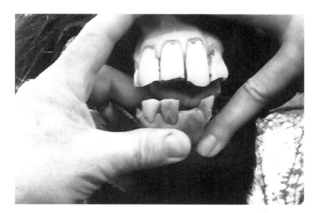

Figure 8-16. Missing incisor. (*Courtesy Tami Mitz, Brenham, TX.*)

Missing or Malpositioned Incisors

If an incisor is missing, the opposing tooth elongates, impeding lateral excursion of the mandible and eventually putting pressure on the mucosa and bone of the opposite jaw (Fig. 8-16). The overlong tooth must be reduced periodically to avoid these problems.

Malerupted or otherwise malpositioned incisors are not in full occlusion. As a result, part or all of the tooth elongates because it is not being worn normally by the opposing tooth. The overgrown tooth (or the elongated portion) should be reduced periodically to optimize lateral excursion. If the malocclusion is severe, it may be best to extract the tooth. In either case, the opposing tooth should also be addressed.

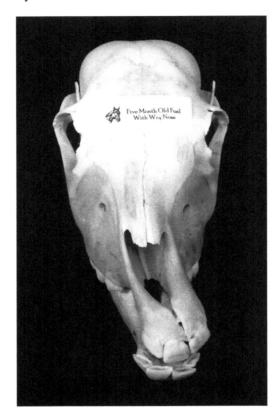

Figure 8-17. Wry mouth skull. (*Courtesy Tami Mitz, Brenham, TX.*)

Wry Mouth

Wry mouth and wry nose are more common in minis than in larger breeds. The defect ranges from subtle (e.g., malalignment of a single incisor) to severe (e.g., deviation of the entire incisor arcade by up to 60 degrees). Dental care for minis with wry mouth or wry nose basically involves reducing the incisor arcades as necessary to optimize lateral excursion and, if necessary, extracting unopposed incisors. Shear mouth (see Chapter 5) is common in horses with wry mouth or wry nose. Frequent dental care is required to maintain quality of life in these horses (Figs. 8-17 and 8-18).

Siamese Teeth

Occasionally, two deciduous incisors are fused, like "Siamese" twins. When the time comes for one of the deciduous incisors to be shed, it is necessary to separate the two teeth to allow development and eruption of the permanent incisors to proceed normally. Separating the fused incisors is easily done with a diamond cutting wheel (Fig. 8-19).

CANINES

Owing to the small size of the head in minis, the location of the canines can vary considerably. Some erupt immediately behind the 3s, as though they're part of the incisor arcade; in fact, the upper and lower canines may even be in occlusion. In other cases the canines erupt medially and grow toward the midline. Because these teeth can irritate, damage, or otherwise interfere with the tongue, they must be reduced nearly to the gum line and kept very smooth.

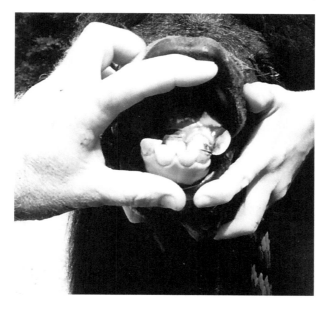

Figure 8-18. Wry mouth. (*Courtesy Tami Mitz, Brenham, TX.*)

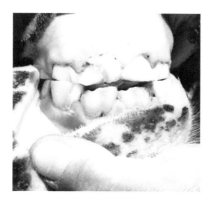

Figure 8-19. Siamese teeth. (*Courtesy Tami Mitz, Brenham, TX.*)

WOLF TEETH

The wolf teeth in minis can be quite large. In some cases they are so large and so long that they resemble upper 6 hooks at first glance. These wolf teeth should be extracted to prevent interference with rostro-caudal movement and lateral excursion of the mandible. In other instances, a good general rule to follow is that the wolf teeth should be removed whenever they are large and space is an issue. As in larger breeds, wolf tooth extraction is commonly performed in minis that must wear a bit (Fig. 8-20).

CHEEK TEETH

Eruption Cysts and Cap Extraction

Owing to the small size and refined shape of the head, mandibular or maxillary swellings associated with eruption of the permanent cheek teeth (eruption cysts) are very common in young minis (Color Plates 64 and 65). Removal of the deciduous premolars (caps) may be required to encourage eruption of the permanent tooth and reduction of the eruption cyst in show animals. However, *it is very important to know the exact age of the horse* before removing any of the deciduous premolars. Premature removal of the deciduous premolar can damage the developing permanent tooth.

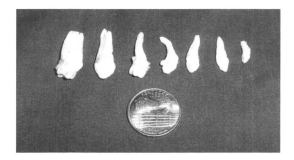

Figure 8-20. Wolf teeth in minis can be quite large. (*Courtesy Tami Mitz, Brenham, TX.*)

Eruption cysts often appear as early as 2 years of age. However, deciduous premolars must not be extracted this early. When the owner insists that something be done, slightly reducing the height of the deciduous 6s and 7s may decrease the size of the eruption cysts (by relieving pressure on the unerupted permanent teeth) until the caps can be safely extracted. The 6s and 7s are reduced in height by approximately 1 mm such that a 2-mm gap is created between the upper and lower arcades. A small rotary burr works well for this procedure. The same approach can be taken with the deciduous 8s in 3- and 4-year-olds.

As a general rule of thumb, the deciduous 6s can be safely extracted once the upper deciduous 1s have been shed (typically at around 3 years of age). The deciduous 7s can usually be safely extracted 3 months later. The deciduous 8s can be safely extracted once the upper deciduous 2s have been shed (typically at around 4 years of age).

However, no deciduous premolar should be extracted unless it is found to be loose. In most cases there is no obvious line of demarcation between the cap and the emerging permanent tooth, so it is necessary to palpate or manipulate the cap with forceps to determine whether it can safely be extracted. If the cap can be wiggled easily, it can be safely extracted.

It is important to bear in mind that eruption times in minis can be highly variable. Some horses are 12 months behind the "norm" for this breed, meaning that they do not even begin shedding any deciduous teeth until they are 4 years old!

Maleruptions and Malocclusions

Overcrowding of the molar arcades is common in minis and results in a variety of maleruptions and malocclusions. In some cases one or more teeth erupt lingual or palatal to the arcade. In other cases, malocclusion results in chisel-shaped teeth that ulcerate the buccal mucosa (Fig. 8-21). In extreme situations, overcrowding causes the upper 11s to impinge on the orbit (Fig. 8-22).

It is relatively common for malpositioned or maloccluded teeth to migrate and become loosened. Reshaping or reducing the abnormal portion of the tooth generally does not prevent the tooth from loosening nor restore its periodontal attachment. When the tooth is loose, it should be extracted. The following discussion describes some specific abnormalities that are often encountered in miniature horse dentistry.

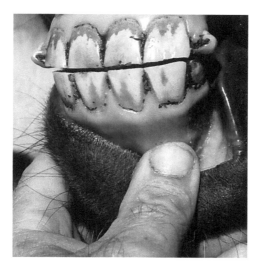

Figure 8-21. In other cases, malocclusion results in chisel-shaped teeth that ulcerate the buccal mucosa. (*Courtesy Tami Mitz, Brenham, TX.*)

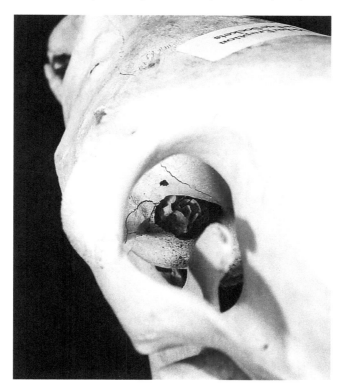

Figure 8-22. In extreme situations, overcrowding causes the upper 11s to impinge on the orbit. (*Courtesy Tami Mitz, Brenham, TX.*)

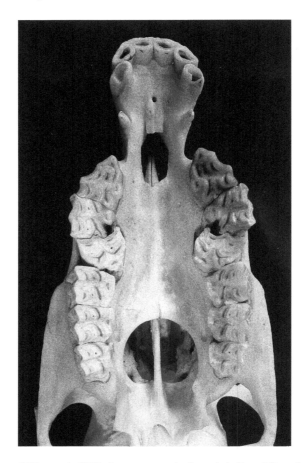

Figure 8-23. The 108 and 208 have erupted palatally. (*Courtesy Tami Mitz, Brenham, TX.*)

Malerupted Upper 8s

Because space is at a premium in the molar arcades, it is common for a permanent upper 8 (108 or 208) to malerupt in such a way that the deciduous 8 is retained and the permanent tooth erupts palatal to the deciduous tooth (Fig. 8-23). The deciduous tooth can irritate the buccal mucosa (because the cap is often pushed buccally by the erupting permanent tooth), and the permanent tooth can interfere with the tongue. In some cases a facial draining tract develops over the buccally displaced deciduous tooth.

To correct this problem, the deciduous tooth must be extracted so the permanent tooth can migrate into a more normal position. Extraction of the deciduous tooth is easily accomplished by using an elevator to separate the gingiva from the tooth, then using molar or cap extractors to remove the tooth. If necessary, the permanent tooth can be used as a fulcrum.

Until the permanent 8 migrates laterally into the arcade, it may need to be shortened and/or rounded so that it does not interfere with the tongue. If removal of the deciduous 8 leaves a void on the buccal side of the arcade, the buccal portions of the permanent 6 and 7 can be reduced to prevent feed material from packing into the space left by the deciduous 8.

Occasionally there is insufficient space in the molar arcade for the permanent 8 to migrate into its normal position, despite removal of the deciduous 8. When this situation occurs, the permanent 8 remains malpositioned and in need of either frequent reduction or extraction (Color Plate 66).

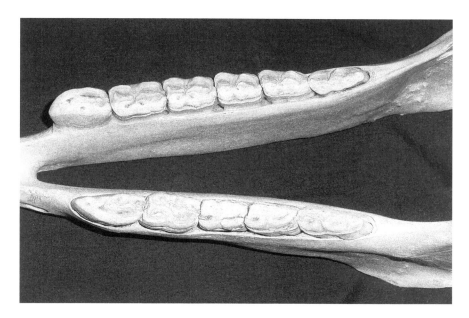

Figure 8-24. Some small minis have only five cheek teeth in the lower arcades and six in the uppers. (*Courtesy Tami Mitz, Brenham, TX.*)

Overgrown Upper 8s

With this malocclusion, a space between the lower 7 and lower 8 allows a portion of the upper 8 to elongate; often the overgrown portion of the tooth is V-shaped. In most, but not all cases, the gap in the lower arcade closes once the overgrown portion of the upper 8 is reduced. Reduction is best performed with a rotary burr. Molar cutters should not be used; not only is fracture of the tooth a possibility, but the shape of the tooth makes it difficult to reduce the overlong portion with this instrument.

Overgrown 11s

Some small minis have only five cheek teeth in the lower arcades and six in the uppers. The opposite can also occur, in which there are only five cheek teeth in the upper arcades and six in the lowers. This problem may occur on only one side of the mouth or on both the left and right sides. In any case, the unopposed 11s become overgrown (Fig. 8-24).

A full-mouth speculum is essential for identifying and correcting this problem. Because access to the 11s is extremely limited in these small patients, molar cutters may be the best instruments for reducing the overlong portions of the 11s. Some of these teeth are so long that it is impossible to see or feel the "occlusal" surface of the tooth, making it very difficult to reduce them using a burr.

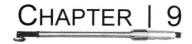

CHAPTER 9

Continuing Education

Scott K. Greene

Among the most important obligations of any practitioner are these: to acquire greater knowledge, to expand his or her skills, and to improve the standard of patient care and client service provided. Continuing education (CE) is the key to meeting these obligations. In the past 10 to 15 years, the field of equine dentistry has seen significant changes and dramatic advances in instrumentation and techniques. Fortunately, CE opportunities for veterinarians and equine dental technicians have expanded concurrently. These opportunities include lectures and hands-on instruction at conferences and equine dentistry workshops, technical support and structured training by equipment manufacturers, textbooks, journal articles, Internet discussion groups, and one-on-one interactions with more experienced colleagues.

Horse owners and trainers are becoming well educated regarding proper dental care and the potential benefit for their horses. They expect their veterinarian to provide those services or refer them to a qualified practitioner. In most patients, "knocking off a few sharp points" is not considered proper equine dentistry. CE can be expensive and time-consuming. However, Derek Bok, former president of Harvard University, encapsulated the importance of CE when he said, "If you think education is expensive, try ignorance" (Color Plate 67).

MOTORIZED INSTRUMENTS

Education and training are particularly important in the use of motorized dental instruments. An improperly educated, inexperienced individual can rapidly compromise the dental arcades or cause significant oral trauma. Proper use of these instruments requires that the practitioner (1) is familiar with the diversity of oral pathologic conditions in equine patients, (2) understands what is appropriate for crown height and occlusal surface angle, (3) learns about the different instruments and techniques that can be used to restore the arcades, and (4) is aware of the potential complications associated with the use of these instruments.

It is imperative that any person entering the horse's oral cavity with motorized instruments have a thorough understanding of the fundamentals of proper dentistry. Most practical teaching laboratories have instruments available and experienced practitioners to instruct on their proper use.

NEW AND ADVANCED TECHNIQUES

Equine dentistry is a dynamic discipline. New procedures are continually being developed, and advanced techniques are becoming more commonplace as information and ideas are disseminated among equine dental practitioners (Color Plate 68). Examples include the treatment of periodontal disease, endodontics, and composite restoration of decayed teeth. Although intraoral extractions are routinely performed by practitioners in the field, the time has come when preservation of the diseased tooth is a primary focus.

Innovative companies and individuals continue to modify instruments and adapt techniques that have proven effective in preventing tooth loss in small animal and human dentistry. These advancements are exciting, and will enable equine practitioners and technicians to provide a higher level of patient care.

CONTINUING EDUCATION RESOURCES

Books

Several equine dental texts have been published in recent years, including the following:
- Equine Dentistry: The Theory and Practice of Equine Dental Maintenance by D. Jeffrey, published by World Wide Equine, Inc., Glenns Ferry, Idaho, 1996
- Oral Biomechanics and Dental Equilibration in Equidae by D. Jeffrey, published by World Wide Equine, Inc., Glenns Ferry, Idaho, 1998
- Dentistry, edited by E.M. Gaughan and R.M. DeBowes, Veterinary Clinics of North America—Equine Practice, 14:2, published by W.B. Saunders, Philadelphia, Pennsylvania, 1998
- Equine Dentistry, edited by G.J. Baker and K.J. Easley, published by W.B. Saunders, Philadelphia, Pennsylvania, 1999
- Equine Dentistry: A Practical Guide by P. Pence, published by Lippincott Williams & Wilkins, Philadelphia, Pennsylvania, 2002

For anyone interested in the history of equine dentistry, Dr. Louis Merillat's text *Animal Dentistry and Diseases of the Mouth* (Alexander Egar, Chicago, 1906) provides a fascinating glimpse of equine dentistry 100 years ago.[*]

Periodicals

Although there currently is no veterinary journal devoted solely to equine dentistry, articles on this subject appear from time to time in the following veterinary publications:
- Equine Veterinary Journal
- Equine Veterinary Education
- Compendium on Continuing Education for the Practicing Veterinarian
- Veterinary Record
- Journal of Veterinary Dentistry
- Equine Practice
- Large Animal Practice

The databases Agricola, CAB Abstracts, and Medline can be used to search these and other publications for articles on specific dentistry topics. Medline can be accessed via the Internet at PubMed (www.ncbi.nlm.nih.gov). However, Medline archives only some of the journals in the previous list.

Other Internet sites at which you may search for published information on equine dentistry include Iknowledgenow (www.iknowledgenow.com), Institute for Scientific Information (www.isinet.com), and International Veterinary Information Service (www.ivis.org).

In addition to the previously listed journals, World Wide Equine, Inc., publishes the *Horse Dentistry and Bitting Journal.*

Conferences, Seminars, and Workshops

Options for acquiring equine dentistry CE are more diverse and accessible than ever before. Equine dentistry continues to be one of the most requested topics for veterinary conferences, seminars, and workshops, so CE opportunities are plentiful. Check with your national, state, regional, and special interest veterinary groups for upcoming meetings that include equine dentistry topics. These meetings can provide formal (classroom) instruction, practical (hands-on) training, and reference materials (e.g., proceedings and notes). They also allow the practitioner the opportunity to interact with presenters for one-on-one discussion and tutelage.

The American Association of Equine Practitioners (AAEP)† frequently includes equine dentistry topics in the scientific program at its annual convention. The AAEP now publishes the proceedings of the annual conventions on CD-ROM, enabling easy access to articles from previous years.

Veterinary Colleges

Veterinary colleges are increasingly providing formal and practical instruction in equine dentistry for veterinary students, veterinarians, and horse owners. Several universities have expanded their curricula, offer elective short courses, and invite experienced practitioners to provide instruction on equine dentistry to faculty members and students. Many practitioners and university professors have put forth a concerted effort to increase the amount of equine dentistry instruction available to veterinary students and technicians. These clinicians should be commended for the positive impact their efforts have had on college curricula.

Equine Dentistry Organizations and Companies

The following organizations or companies also provide various CE opportunities for veterinarians, animal health technicians, equine dental technicians, and horse owners:
- Academy of Equine Dentistry*
- American School of Equine Dentistry†
- Equi-Dent Technologies, Inc.‡
- International Association of Equine Dentistry§
- Pacific Equine Dental Institute‖
- Veterinary Dental Forum¶

The Academy of Veterinary Dentistry# has recently established a 2-year equine pathway for Fellowship in the Academy.

Internet Discussion Groups

An Internet community, horsedentistry@yahoogroups.com, provides practitioners an opportunity to share opinions on particular cases, as well as discuss other subjects related to equine dentistry. The site is visited by an international group of veterinarians, veterinary technicians, and equine dental technicians.

The Equine Clinician's Network (ECN, join-ecn@listserve.vetmed.wsu.edu) provides equine veterinarians an opportunity to share insights regarding equine medicine and surgery. Dentistry is a relatively frequent, usually stimulating, and always enlightening topic. This listserve, which is composed of an international group of veterinarians, allows practitioners to interact with an experienced and generous group of colleagues, several of whom have a special interest in equine dentistry.

Colleagues

Practitioners should take advantage of any opportunity to spend time with colleagues who share their interest in equine dentistry. I have never watched or worked with another practitioner without acquiring some new gems of information. Take every opportunity to share case reports and learn what others have found to be effective treatment options, techniques to be avoided, and potential outcomes and prognoses. If presented with the opportunity, write or co-author an article, submit an abstract, or publish a case report. Strive to continue the dissemination of equine dental information among your colleagues.

SUMMARY

Those involved in providing or receiving dentistry-related CE appreciate the current interest in the topic, and practitioners all appreciate that they will always have more to learn. As a Princeton freshman in 1933, Albert Einstein wrote, "Never regard your study as a duty, but as the enviable opportunity to learn, to know the liberating influence of beauty in the realm of the spirit for your own personal joy and to the profit of the community to which your later work belongs."

*Available from Harlton's Equine Specialties, 792 Olenhurst Court, Columbus, OH 43235-2163 or from www.harltons.com.

†American Association of Equine Practitioners, 4075 Iron Works Pkwy, Lexington, KY 40511, www.aaep.org.

*Academy of Equine Dentistry, PO Box 999, Glenns Ferry, ID 83623, www.equinedentistry.com.

†American School of Equine Dentistry, PO Box 126, Brunswick, MD 21716, www.amscheqdentistry.com.

‡Equi-Dent Technologies, Inc, PO Box 5877, Sparks, NV 89432, www.equi-dent.com.

§ International Association of Equine Dentistry, PO Box 2458, Brevard, NC 28712, www.iaedglobal.org.

‖Pacific Equine Dental Institute, 34730 Glacier Ave, St Helens, OR 97051.

¶Veterinary Dental Forum, 200 Forth Avenue, Suite 900, Nashville, TN 37219.

#Academy of Veterinary Dentistry, www.avdonline.org.

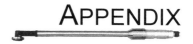

Dental Suppliers

Academy of Equine Dentistry P.O. Box 999 Glenns Ferry, ID 83623 208-366-2315 www.equinedentalacademy.com *Continuing education, books, and publications*

Advanced Equine Dentistry 6101 Katz Road Grass Lake, MI 49240 888-372-1069 *Dentistry posters, brochures, and flip charts*

Alberts Equine Dental Supply, Inc. Box 11-184 Loudonville, NY 12211 877-336-8258 www.alberts.net *Dental instruments, equipment, and supplies*

Capps Manufacturing, Inc. 4894 West Birch Rd. Clatonia, NE 68328 888-881-4686 www.cappsmanufacturing.com

Carbide Products 22711 Western Ave. Torrance, CA 90501 888-64-BLADE www.horsedental.com *Dental equipment, instruments, and supplies*

D&B Equine Enterprises, Inc. 207 Silverhill Way N.W. Calgary, Alberta, Canada T3B 4K9 877-969-2233 www.powerfloat.net *PowerFloat and supplies*

Dr. Allen's Horse Dentistry Attention: Dawn Route 1 Box 176E Patterson, MO 63956 888-603-9689 www.horsedentist.com facticiouspressink@semo.net *Dental charts, posters, and brochures*

DW Tooling RR #1, Box 3090 Castle Dr. Leechburg, PA 15656 866-4DWTOOL dwtool@nauticom.net

Equi-Dent Technologies 715 Greenbrae Dr. Sparks, NV 89431 775-358-6695 www.equi-dent.com *Instruments, supplies, continuing education, and dental charts*

Franck's Pharmacy 202 SW 17th St. Ocala, FL 34474 877-892-9991 www.francks.com *Supplier for Yohimbine and Naloxone*

Harlton's Equine Dental Specialties, Inc. 792 Olenhurst Court Columbus, OH 43235-2163 800-247-3901 www.harltons.com *Dental equipment and supplies*

Jupiter Veterinary Products 3635 North 6th St. Harrisburg, PA 17110 717-233-4004 www.jupitervetproducts.com *Veterinary and dental equipment, instruments, and supplies*

Light Tech 8900 W. Josephine Rd. Sebring, FL 33875 800-462-5542 www.light-tech.com *Halogen headlights*

Milburn Distributions, Inc. P.O. Box 42810 Phoenix, AZ 85080 800-279-6452 *Dental equipment, instruments, and supplies*

Olsen & Silk Abrasives P.O. Box 8467 Salem, MA 01970 978-744-4720 regritme@aol.com *Dental instruments, equipment, supplies, and service*

Pacific Equine Dental Institute 7118 Cinnamon Teal Way El Dorado Hills, CA 95762 800-241-3079 www.equine_dentistry.net *Periodontal equipment, supplies, and continuing education*

Promax Equine Dental 3352A Coffey Lane Santa Rosa, CA 95403 800-933-1562 sales@promaxequinedental.com *Instruments, blades, burs, and cut-off wheels*

Rayovac Corporation P.O. Box 44960 Madison, WI 53744-4960 608-275-3340 consumers@rayovac.com *Belt battery pack model*

Rena's Equine Dental Instruments 4055 Casa Blanca Reno, NV 89502 877-912-7122 www.equinedentalinstrument.com *Equine dental instruments, supplies, continuing education, and dental charts*

Richard O. Miller DVM–IAED/Ex 23411 Via Alondra Coto de Caza, CA 92679 949-858-1975 richdent@juno.com *DataDent (equine dental evaluation and charting software program)*

Sontec Instruments 7248 South Tucson Way Englewood, CO 80112 800-821-7496 *Equine dental instruments*

Spencer's Equine Services, Inc. 6625 Calvin Lee Road Groveland, FL 34736 352-429-8207 MOUTHSPECULUM1@cs.com *Full mouth speculum*

Stubbs Equine Innovations, Inc. HC3 Box 38 Johnson City, TX 78636 830-868-9363 www.stubbs-equi.com *Dental equipment, instruments, and supplies*

SwissVet Veterinary Products 1952 Lee Rd. 65 Auburn, AL 36830 877-794-7735 www.swissvet.com *Dental equipment*

T.R. Cherry & Co., Inc. Route 4, Box 319C Loogootee, IN 47553 812-295-2482 www.equident.com *Equine dental equipment*

Western Instrument Co. 4950 York St. Denver, CO 80216 800-525-2065 www.westerninstrument.com *Dental equipment, instruments, and supplies*

World Wide Equine P.O. Box 1040 Glenns Ferry, ID 83623 800-331-5485 www.horsedentistry.com *Dental instruments and supplies*

*Page numbers followed by f indicate figures; b indicates boxes.**